The Body in the Mind

The Body in the Mind

Exercise Addiction, Body Image, and the Use of Enhancement Drugs

Edited by

Ornella Corazza
Department of Clinical, Pharmaceutical and Biological Sciences, University of Hertfordshire, UK
Department of Psychology and Cognitive Science, University of Trento, Italy

Artemisa Rocha Dores
School of Health, Polytechnic Institute of Porto, Portugal
Laboratory of Neuropsychophysiology, Faculty of Psychology and Education Sciences,
University of Porto, Portugal

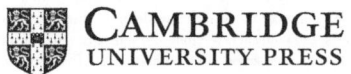

CAMBRIDGE
UNIVERSITY PRESS

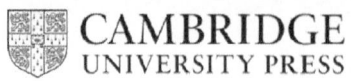

Shaftesbury Road, Cambridge CB2 8EA, United Kingdom

One Liberty Plaza, 20th Floor, New York, NY 10006, USA

477 Williamstown Road, Port Melbourne, VIC 3207, Australia

314–321, 3rd Floor, Plot 3, Splendor Forum, Jasola District Centre,
New Delhi – 110025, India

103 Penang Road, #05–06/07, Visioncrest Commercial, Singapore 238467

Cambridge University Press is part of Cambridge University Press & Assessment,
a department of the University of Cambridge.

We share the University's mission to contribute to society through the pursuit of
education, learning and research at the highest international levels of excellence.

www.cambridge.org
Information on this title: www.cambridge.org/9781911623724

DOI: 10.1017/9781911623731

First published 2023

A catalogue record for this publication is available from the British Library.

Library of Congress Cataloging-in-Publication Data
Names: Corazza, Ornella, author. | Dores, Artemisa Rocha, author.
Title: The body in the mind : exercise addiction, body image and the use of
    enhancement drugs / Ornella Corazza, Artemisa Rocha Dores.
Description: New York : Cambridge University Press, 2023. | Includes index.
Identifiers: LCCN 2023000072 (print) | LCCN 2023000073 (ebook) |
    ISBN 9781911623724 (paperback) | ISBN 9781911623731 (epub)
Subjects: LCSH: Exercise addiction. | Body image disturbance.
Classification: LCC RC569.5.E94 C67 2023 (print) | LCC RC569.5.E94 (ebook) |
    DDC 616.85/2–dc23/eng/20230125
LC record available at https://lccn.loc.gov/2023000072
LC ebook record available at https://lccn.loc.gov/2023000073

ISBN 978-1-911-62372-4 Paperback

To Gioia Corazza and all the children who, like her, have the right to grow up in a world free of constraints and addictions.

Contents

Figures

Tables

Boxes

Contributors

Manuel Alcaraz-Ibáñez, PhD,
Health Research Centre and
Department of Education, University
of Almería, Spain

Giuseppe Bersani, MD, Department
of Medico-Surgical Sciences and
Biotechnologies, Sapienza University
of Rome, Italy

**Thomas Brosnan, MSc, MBACP,
FDAP,** Department of Applied
Science, London South Bank
University, UK

Kate Brown, BSc, MSc, MCSP,
Cambridgeshire and
Peterborough NHS Foundation
Trust, UK

Julius Burkauskas, PhD, Laboratory
of Behavioral Medicine, Lithuanian
University of Health Sciences,
Lithuania

Irene P. Carvalho, PhD, Clinical
Neurosciences and Mental Health
Department and CINTESIS, University
of Porto, Portugal

**Valeria Catalani, MSc, PhD
Student,** Psychopharmacology,
Drug Misuse and Novel Psychoactive
Substances Research Unit, University
of Hertfordshire, UK

Franca Ceci, MD, Department of
Neuroscience, Imaging and Clinical
Sciences, University G. d'Annunzio of
Chieti-Pescara, Italy

**Martin Chandler, BSc, MSc, PGCE,
PhD,** School of Sport, Exercise and
Rehabilitation Sciences, University of
Birmingham, UK

Dorotea Cicconcelli, MD,
Department of Clinical, Pharmaceutical
and Biological Sciences, University of
Hertfordshire, UK

Ornella Corazza, PhD, Department
of Clinical, Pharmaceutical and
Biological Sciences, University of
Hertfordshire, UK

**Andrea Corbett, BSc,
PGCE,** Transformational Life Coach
and Resilience Practitioner; British
Champion of Women's Physique
and International Figure
Bodybuilder

Ilaria De Luca, MD, Department of
Clinical, Pharmaceutical and
Biological Sciences, University of
Hertfordshire, UK

Merve Denizci Nazlıgül, PhD,
Clinical Psychologist, Turkey

**Francesco Di Carlo, MD, PhD
Student,** Department of
Neuroscience, Imaging and Clinical
Sciences, University G. d'Annunzio of
Chieti-Pescara, Italy

Massimo Di Giannantonio, PhD,
Department of Neuroscience, Imaging
and Clinical Sciences, University
G. d'Annunzio of Chieti-Pescara, Italy

Artemisa Rocha Dores, BSc, MSc, PhD, Center for Rehabilitation Research, School of Health, Polytechnic Institute of Porto, Portugal; Laboratory of Neuropsychophysiology, Faculty of Psychology and Education Sciences, University of Porto, Portugal

Alice C. English, MSc, INS Istituto di Neuroscienze, Italy

Hironobu Fujiwara, MD, PhD, Department of Neuropsychiatry, University of Kyoto, Japan; Artificial Intelligence Ethics and Society Team, RIKEN Center for Advanced Intelligence Project, Japan

Valentina Giorgetti, MD, Department of Clinical, Pharmaceutical and Biological Sciences, University of Hertfordshire, UK

Mark D. Griffiths, PhD, Psychology Department, Nottingham Trent University, UK

Oluyinka Idowu, MBBS, MSc, Dip. RSA, MCIPD, Pg.Cert SWP, PGCE, SFHEA, PTLLS, Department of Clinical, Pharmaceutical and Biological Sciences, University of Hertfordshire, UK

Konstantinos Ioannidis, MD, MSc, AFHEA, MRCPsych, PhD, Cambridgeshire and Peterborough NHS Foundation Trust, UK; Department of International Health, Care and Public Health Research Institute, Maastricht University, Netherlands; Department of Psychiatry, University of Cambridge, UK

Jim McVeigh, RGN, MSc, PhD, Substance Use and Associated Behaviours Research Group, Manchester Metropolitan University, UK

Giovanni Martinotti, MD, PhD, Department of Neuroscience, Imaging and Clinical Sciences, University G. d'Annunzio of Chieti-Pescara, Italy; Department of Clinical, Pharmaceutical and Biological Sciences, University of Hertfordshire, UK

Roisin Mooney, BSc, PhD, Department of Psychiatry, University of Oxford, UK

Pedro Morgado, MD, PhD, Life and Health Sciences Research Institute, School of Medicine, University of Minho, Portugal; Department of Psychiatry, Hospital de Braga, Portugal

Attilio Negri, MD, Department of Clinical, Pharmaceutical and Biological Sciences, University of Hertfordshire, UK

Stefano Pallanti, MD, PhD, Montefiore Medical Center, Albert Einstein College of Medicine, USA; INS Istituto di Neuroscienze, Italy

Adrian Paterna, MA, PhD, Health Research Centre and Department of Education, University of Almería, Spain

Silvia Rossato, MD, Dual Diagnosis Unit, Clinica Parco dei Tigli, Italy

Angela Scoppettone, MD, Dual Diagnosis Unit, Clinica Parco dei Tigli, Italy

Mami Shibata, MD, Department of Neuropsychiatry, University of Kyoto, Japan

Álvaro Sicilia, PhD, Health Research Centre and Department of Education, University of Almería, Spain

Pierluigi Simonato, MD, PhD, Dual Diagnosis Unit, Clinica Parco dei Tigli, Italy; Department of Clinical, Pharmaceutical and Biological Sciences, University of Hertfordshire, UK

Charlotte Taylor, BSc, MSc, Department of Clinical Psychology, University of East Anglia and Norfolk and Suffolk NHS Foundation Trust, UK

Anna Tippett, MSc, PhD, School of Law, University of Hertfordshire, UK

Honor D. Townshend, MSc, PhD Candidate School of Law, University of Hertfordshire, UK Royal Docks School of Business and Law, University of East London, UK

Gemma Anne Yarwood, BSc, MEd, PGCE, PhD, Substance Use and Associated Behaviours Research Group, Manchester Metropolitan University, UK

Acknowledgements

This book was written during a very challenging time for humanity, due to the COVID-19 pandemic. We are deeply grateful to all the co-authors of this book, who – despite the widespread suffering, loss of loved ones, increased workloads, and necessity for social distancing – felt the need to come together to share their knowledge and experience of body image and related psychopathological issues that they had observed among their patients.

In particular, we would like to thank Dr Dorotea Cicconcelli for supporting us with the editing of this book with such determination and accuracy. Highly capable and committed young scholars such as herself are urgently needed, and we wish her every success in her promising career as a clinical psychologist. In addition, we would like to thank Mariana Machado and Valter Costa for their help with editorial tasks during the last phase of the project.

We would also like to thank Professor Henrietta Bowden-Jones for proposing the original idea for this book, and Maria Filopoulou for providing such an inspirational cover design. The *Underwater Swimmers III* represents to us the ultimate expression of freedom of the human body when in harmony with nature – a body that is free from societal constraints and harmful addictions.

Finally, we owe a debt of gratitude to the team at Cambridge University Press for their untiring interest in, attention to, and advice on our manuscript. It has been a long but enriching journey.

We are thankful to you all.

Ornella Corazza
Artemisa Rocha Dores
20 November 2022

Introduction

We live in an image-focused society that places a heavy emphasis on striving for perfection. Individuals are exposed to constant pressure regarding their appearance, both from the beauty and fitness industry and through social media. In this context, fitness is increasingly viewed as a means to get in shape, look good, and achieve a certain aesthetic ideal, rather than a way to improve health and performance. 'Train, Eat, Sleep, Repeat', 'Don't stop until you're proud', 'The pain you feel today will be the strength you feel tomorrow', and 'No pain, no gain' are just a few examples of 'fitspirational' quotes that are used to inspire a healthy lifestyle through exercise.

In parallel, technological developments have led to a new set of values, behaviours, and means of sharing advice on products, specialist diets, and other techniques designed to enhance physical appearance. Every day, millions of texts and selfies are posted on social media, promoting the visual representation of ostensibly fit and healthy bodies. This context of 'aesthetic idealization' constitutes fertile ground for the development of exercise addiction alongside other disorders, such as body dysmorphic disorder, eating disorders, and related psychopathologies.

In this book, through a combination of personal accounts, clinical cases, and exploration of the dominant scientific explanations, we present a contemporary perspective on exercise addiction, designed to shed new light on these rapidly emerging trends in society, which are strongly interlinked with the desire both to appear to have and to actually possess a 'perfect' body. We prioritise here the identification and analysis of behaviours among those at risk of addiction, who rarely come to the attention of health professionals, in part because they do not consider themselves 'addicted' in the traditional sense, and in part due to the normalization of their behaviour by society. Often, if care is sought, primary care doctors, fitness coaches, and others are consulted, rather than psychiatrists or psychologists.

In this book we explore how such a concern about physical appearance could act as a precursor to, or be symptomatic of, not only exercise addiction, but also other underlying and potentially underdiagnosed clinical conditions and mood disorders, as well as the use of image- and performance-enhancing drugs (IPEDs), with potentially damaging consequences for health and well-being. The term 'IPEDs' is used here as an umbrella term to include a wide range of new drugs that can alter the functions of the body and enhance muscle growth, reduce body fat, and promote weight loss [1,2]. Although IPEDs have been in circulation for some years, particularly anabolic-androgenic steroids (AAS), which are most commonly used by athletes and bodybuilders [3], the availability of these drugs on the Internet has increased their accessibility and thus led to greater consumption by wider society. Often advertised via social media platforms as 'natural,' 'healthier', and 'safer' alternatives to medicines, IPEDs attract the attention of vulnerable individuals who want to enhance their bodies – in order to look stronger, younger, and more beautiful – more quickly than can be achieved by natural means. Driven by the false perception that 'natural equals healthy', they might be unaware that some ingredients (listed or otherwise) could include undisclosed biologically active compounds that could expose them to a range of health risks, such as allergic reactions, liver damage, mercury poisoning, brain damage, or even risk of death. Vulnerable individuals, especially those who are unhappy with their body or its abilities, are most likely to purchase and use such substances, and such hazardous behaviour might be symptomatic of body dysmorphic disorder, characterized by a distressing and disabling preoccupation with perceived flaws in one's appearance that are not observable to others, and by other psychopathologies, such as exercise addiction and poor mental health [4].

This book addresses major knowledge gaps, and identifies areas where there is a need to develop new interventions in the field, in order to improve the mental health and well-being both of those affected and of their families. It is designed primarily for clinicians, researchers, practitioners, and graduate students with an interest in the fields of addiction, body image, and substance misuse, in order to improve understanding of the conceptual underpinnings, aetiologies, prevention methods, and treatments available. In addition, the book presents an unprecedented collection of case studies drawn from the populations who are most affected, including frequent exercisers, psychiatric patients, and people with eating disorders. By highlighting their patterns of drug consumption and their underlying psychopathological conditions, we aim to facilitate a better understanding of the underlying risks, while contributing to the improvement of clinical practice, and encouraging innovative prevention responses to behaviours for which the boundaries between normal and pathological are often blurred. Each chapter includes references to the latest scientific literature with regard to typical symptoms, classification, aetiology, and assessment, making this book a valuable resource for the professional development of those involved in medical research, sports psychology, health promotion, public health, social work, and health education.

For maximum clarity, the book has been divided into three core sections.

Section 1, titled 'From Exercise to Addiction: An Introduction to the Phenomenon', consists of a range of chapters about the 'dark' side of exercise. Although physical exercise has a variety of well-recognized health benefits (e.g., improved quality of life, body functioning, muscular strength, and endurance, decreased fatigue, lower incidence of cardiovascular disease and type 2 diabetes, and reduced risk of depression), exercise can also become an addiction. Section 1 reflects on the underlying neurobiological mechanism, and also explains how the emergence of problematic exercising is strongly linked to other behavioural addictions (e.g., pathological gambling, compulsive shopping, and Internet and social media addiction). It highlights the fact that such potentially highly addictive behaviours have not yet been included in the fifth edition of the *Diagnostic and Statistical Manual of Mental Disorders (DSM-5)* [5], which at present only contains gambling as a 'Non-Substance-Related Disorder'. Section 1 of this book argues that a new DSM-5 classification would reflect the increasing interest in this topic and the shift towards a new perspective in which the presence of a psychoactive substance is not a prerequisite for addictive disorders.

Section 2, titled 'Reaching the Extreme with Exercise: A Collection of Clinical Case Studies', presents clinical case studies of people affected by exercise addiction, all written by leading authorities in the field of behavioural addiction and by front-line clinicians. The chapters in this section emphasise the previously unexplored links with other psychopathologies, such as body dysmorphic disorder and eating disorders, as well as the use of IPEDs to improve physical appearance and/or boost performance more rapidly than can be achieved by natural means, and they discuss the commonly unknown underlying risks associated with these behaviours (e.g., contamination of products, safety hazards, potential for injury).

Section 3, titled 'Exploring the Motivations Behind Exercise Addiction', presents a selection of personal accounts written by people who have been actively involved in the sporting environment, and who have agreed to share their views and experiences of problematic exercise. Their testimonies provide a unique subjective perspective that will help both to shed new light on the personal motivations underlying compulsive exercising, and to offer a deeper understanding of the boundaries between positive and problematic aspects of exercise, which are often hard to define.

We strongly believe that this book represents a prime example of effective collaboration among individuals from a variety of disciplines and perspectives, who chose to dedicate their time to collectively address these complex issues during a globally challenging time for all humanity – the COVID-19 pandemic. We hope that you will find it a useful and informative resource. Healthy bodies and minds really matter to us, so let us do our best to benefit society and to improve lives.

References

1 Bates G, McVeigh J. *Image and Performance Enhancing Drugs: 2015 Survey Results.* Centre for Public Health, Liverpool John Moores University, 2016. www.ipedinfo .co.uk/resources/downloads/2015%20National%20IPED%20Info%20Survey% 20report.pdf

2 Corazza O, Simonato P, Demetrovics Z et al. The emergence of Exercise Addiction, Body Dysmorphic Disorder, and other image-related psychopathological correlates in fitness settings: a cross sectional study. *PLoS ONE* 2019; 14: e0213060.

3 Evans-Brown M, McVeigh J, Perkins C, Bellis M. *Human Enhancement Drugs: The Emerging Challenges to Public Health.* North West Public Health Observatory, 2012.

4 Veale DMW. Does primary exercise dependence really exist? In: Annet J, Cripps B, Steinberg H, eds. *Exercise Addiction: Motivation for Participation in Sport and Exercise.* British Psychological Society, 1995: 71–5.

5 American Psychiatric Association. *Diagnostic and Statistical Manual of Mental Disorders*, 5th ed. American Psychiatric Association, 2013.

From Exercise to Addiction: An Introduction to the Phenomenon

Exercise Addiction
Evolution and Challenges for Its Recognition as a Clinical Disorder

Álvaro Sicilia, Manuel Alcaraz-Ibáñez, Adrian Paterna, and Mark D. Griffiths

1.1 Introduction

Extensive research has shown that exercise has health benefits for everyone [1]. However, studies have also suggested that a small minority of individuals may experience negative physical and psychological effects, as they may become addicted to exercise and crave it in a similar way to those who are addicted to substances such as alcohol, nicotine, or other drugs [2,3]. Although the possible negative effects of exercise addiction (EA) were first indicated more than 50 years ago [4–7], to date it has never received formal recognition as a mental disorder in the leading clinical manuals [8,9]. In 2013, the fifth edition of the *Diagnostic and Statistical Manual of Mental Disorders (DSM-5)* [8] incorporated gambling disorder along with substance-related disorders, so the title of this chapter in Section II was changed from 'Substance-Related Disorders' to 'Substance-Related and Addictive Disorders'. This new classification appears to be based on new evidence which suggests that addiction is a disorder of the brain's reward system, regardless of whether the system is activated by a behaviour or a substance [10–12].

The DSM-5 only includes gambling as a behavioural addiction, as well as criteria for internet gaming disorder (IGD) as a behavioural addiction within Section III ('Emerging Measures and Models'). This decision was based on the Substance Use Disorder Workgroup's conclusion that there was insufficient evidence to warrant the full inclusion of IGD as an official mental disorder in Section II. However, the new conceptualization of the diagnosis of addiction opens the door for research into other forms of excessive behaviour that can be potentially addictive. Furthermore, another group of repetitive behaviours, including exercise, was not included due to the lack of scientific evidence for establishing the diagnostic criteria and course descriptions needed to identify these behaviours as mental disorders [8]. Therefore, at the time of writing, EA should be considered as a potentially addictive behaviour and not a behavioural addiction – that is, a behavioural condition with a psychiatric entity that requires a diagnosis [13].

The future incorporation of exercise behaviour as an addiction appears to be contingent on the scientific community reaching some degree of consensus on two important questions that research has been addressing in recent decades [14]. First, there is a need to define the phenomenon of EA and establish a clear rationale, supported by sufficient scientific evidence, for the mechanism by which exercise can be shown to be an addiction. Second, an evidence base is needed to determine how to categorize EA in relation to other possible mental disorders, and whether EA should be considered a distinct disorder. Logistically, only when the first question has been answered will we know the relevance of the second one. If no evidence can be found that exercise may have negative consequences additional to those caused by over-training, there would be no need to consider exercise as a potential addiction or the processes relating to the development and maintenance of EA and its relationship with other mental disorders. This chapter describes in detail how these issues have been addressed over the past 50 years, and shows that although there is some consensus on the potential harm that can be caused by exercise, there is no agreement about the criteria and the mechanism of action by which this behaviour can become addictive. This lack of unanimity has limited the definition, measurement, and treatment of EA.

1.2 The Paradox of Exercise Addiction

The overwhelming evidence for the positive effects of exercise has led to campaigns to promote exercise among the general population since the mid-twentieth century. These exercise promotion policies must be understood in the context of the development of welfare states, which have been implemented in developed countries since the Second World War [15]. However, as a larger percentage of the global population has started to exercise regularly, awareness that exercise can also have detrimental effects on some individuals has increased.

The debate about the harmful effects of exercise – and the fact that some people can become addicted to exercise and crave it in a similar way to those who are addicted to psychoactive substances such as alcohol, nicotine, or other drugs [2] – took place in North America in the late 1960s and the 1970s. Darcy Plymire reported a 10-fold increase in the number of regular runners within just one decade in North America in the 1970s [16]. However, what Plymire found most striking was not the notable rise in the number of individuals exercising, but the fact that many of these runners reported running for longer than the average time recommended by institutions for achieving exercise-related health benefits (e.g., improvement in aerobic fitness and cardiac health). This finding suggested that there had to be motivations other than the health benefits highlighted by institutions for spending so much time on this activity. In the context of this debate, the question arises as to when exercise can be considered to be intense and prolonged.

Some scholars have argued that the motivation for runners to engage in long-term activity was more about pursuing human potential or what Abraham Maslow called 'self-actualization' [17]. In fact, in line with positive psychology, terms such as 'optimal experience' or 'peak moments' have been used to describe the positive states of consciousness that many people with a regular exercise regime claim to experience during practice or competition [18,19]. However, in his book titled *Positive Addiction*, William Glasser proposed that a long-distance run of more than an hour could produce a state of euphoria and expansion of the mind which he called 'positive addiction' [20]. By coining this term, Glasser wanted to highlight the beneficial effects of exercise, in contrast to addiction to other behaviours that could have negative consequences.

The use of the term 'addiction' in relation to a behaviour such as exercise, which has long been considered a positive activity, has been controversial. However, Glasser connected exercising for long periods with withdrawal symptoms, and therefore described it as a positive addiction [20]. He formulated his hypothesis by studying individuals who practised transcendental meditation. People who engaged in this practice reported an altered state of consciousness that had allowed them to make decisive choices and improve their lives. If they did not exercise, they reported experiencing withdrawal symptoms such as depression, anxiety, and guilt. Glasser studied the psychology of running, and found that many runners fitted the criteria for positive addiction.

Glasser's conceptualization of EA as a positive addiction [20] was soon called into question. In fact, some researchers had already pointed out at the end of the 1960s that some exercisers continued to train despite the contraindications they showed for doing so [5]. Baekeland reinforced this observation by indicating the difficulty he had experienced in recruiting athletes to an experiment that attempted to assess the effects of exercise deprivation on sleep [4]. Further support came from some psychiatric case studies reported by Morgan, who found that physical exercise could lead not only to physical injury but also to the serious neglect of daily work and/or family responsibilities [6]. Morgan recognized the existence of negative effects of EA, warning about its dangers [6]. Thereafter, negative factors associated with exercise, such as injury, overtraining, and psychological dysfunction, were progressively identified and included in the conceptualization of EA [21,22]. Although the positive effects of exercise are still recognized today, there is a consensus that excessive and uncontrolled exercise can have negative consequences for a minority of individuals.

1.3 Criteria for Exercise Addiction

Historically, the debate about EA was focused on long-distance running, specifically because of the amount of time that some individuals spent exercising [16,23]. Unsurprisingly, therefore, the first signs of EA to be addressed were those that defined the characteristics of exercise (e.g., frequency, duration, intensity). Possible harmful effects of addictive exercise were identified, such as biomedical factors (e.g., withdrawal symptoms, tolerance), mental health problems (e.g., depression, anxiety), and social consequences (e.g., neglect of work, family, or other social obligations).

In view of the evidence of various features and consequences of problematic exercise, there is now reasonable consensus that EA, like other substance addictions, should be defined as a set of cognitive, behavioural, physiological, and psychological characteristics [24,25]. Research has shown such close similarities between addiction to behaviours (such as exercise) and drug dependence [2,12] that EA has been defined as a strong desire for physical activity, to the extent that it may involve a lack of control which is manifested as physiological characteristics (e.g., tolerance, withdrawal symptoms) and/or mental health problems (e.g. anxiety, depression) [24,26]. However, despite the consensus on the multidimensionality of EA, the criteria for its diagnosis are less clear. Several strategies have been adopted to identify the features that define EA, four of which are highlighted here.

The first strategy examined the features of EA inductively, through the informed response of individuals who exercise regularly. For example, after interviewing 56 adult female exercisers, Bamber et al. suggested that EA has two essential features: (i) impaired psychological, social, physical, and/or behavioural functioning of the individual and (ii) lack of abstinence or the experience of withdrawal symptoms, related to a reluctance to modify the type of exercise or an inability to reduce the amount of exercise [27]. In addition, Bamber et al. considered a number of features that may be indicative of EA, such as exercising in secret or lying about the amount of exercise performed, denial that there is a problem with exercise, exercising alone, and the development of tolerance (i.e., increasing volume, frequency, and/or intensity of exercise required over time) [27]. This strategy may be of interest if it is assumed that addictions may have multiple and heterogeneous characteristics and comorbidity [28], as it would then be important to identify the specific characteristics that distinguish EA from other types of behavioural addictions.

The second strategy involves identifying features of EA and relating these to substance dependence. In this context, research has focused on defining EA based on the criteria for substance use that are listed in some of the leading clinical manuals. For example, Hausenblas et al. operationalized EA as a multidimensional maladaptive pattern leading to a clinically significant disability or affliction and manifested by the presence of at least three of the following seven criteria that are listed in the fourth edition of the DSM [24]: (i) *tolerance*, defined either as a need to increase the amount of exercise to achieve the intended effect, or a decrease in the effect with continued use of the same amount of exercise; (ii) *withdrawal*, manifested by either withdrawal symptoms when unable to exercise (e.g., anxiety, moodiness, irritability), or requiring the same (or a similar) amount of exercise to relieve or avoid withdrawal symptoms; (iii) *intention effects* – engaging in larger amounts of exercise, or exercising over a longer time period; (iv) *lack of control* – a persistent desire or unsuccessful attempts to reduce or control the amount of exercise; (v) *time* – a large amount of time is spent engaged in activities involving exercise; (vi) *reduction in other activities* – social, occupational, and/ or recreational activities are reduced or stopped in order to exercise instead; (vii) *continuance* – exercising continually despite awareness that this is causing a persistent psychological or physical problem [29].

The third strategy focuses on adapting the criteria defined for behavioural addictions to the context of exercise. This type of strategy assumes that there are common components that all behavioural addictions share. On the basis of this assumption, Sussman and Sussman conducted an extensive review of the literature on addiction and, after identifying common elements, highlighted the following five essential characteristics that EA would share with any type of behavioural addiction: (i) a high level of commitment to the behaviour in order to obtain the desired effects that it produces, rather than because of the activity itself; (ii) the activity occupies an important place in the individual's life and is prioritized over other activities; (iii) the satisfaction that is experienced during or at the end of the activity leads to a distraction from life's problems, and generates a feeling of happiness; (iv) a lack of control over decision-making about when to stop the activity; (v) the behaviour has negative consequences, which may vary depending on the type of addictive behaviour, but in exercise become more evident over time as individuals cease engaging in other activities and/or spending time with others (e.g., partner, family) [12]. Following this approach, research by Carnes (cited by Griffiths [11]) compared the signs that could be shared by behavioural addiction and substance use disorder, highlighting elements such as a pattern of uncontrolled behaviour, unsuccessful attempts to limit that behaviour, use of the behaviour as an escape mechanism, significant mood changes, and a reduction in other life activities as a consequence of the behaviour [11]. Other authors, such as Brown [30] and Griffiths [31–35], view addictions as comprising several core components. The 'addiction components model' proposed by Griffiths [33] has been used to define EA according to six core criteria for behavioural addiction: (i) *salience* (exercise becomes the most important activity and dominates the other areas of the individual's life); (ii) *mood modification* (a subjective mood-altering experience is reported as a consequence of engaging in exercise); (iii) *tolerance* (a tendency to need to increase the amount of exercise in order to experience the desired mood-modifying effects); (iv) *withdrawal* (an unpleasant feeling caused by stopping or drastically reducing exercise); (v) *conflict* (exercise being prioritized over other educational and/or occupational activities and interpersonal relationships, and intra-psychic conflict, where the individual knows they should cut down the amount of exercise they are doing but is unable to do so, and experiences a subjective loss of control; (vi) *relapse* (a tendency to repeat the same exercise patterns after a certain time without engaging in exercise).

The fourth strategy involves trying to identify and define features of EA in relation to other associated disorders. The most important example of this strategy is represented by the view that EA is primarily a behaviour used to maintain body weight and shape (e.g., to lose weight) [36–39]. Although the authors of these studies suggest that EA has similar features to substance use disorder and other forms of behavioural addiction (e.g., withdrawal symptoms), they acknowledge that additional features need to be defined to characterize EA in terms of the main disorder from which it is derived. Hence the use of exercise as a form of weight control, the rigid behavioural pattern, and the positive reinforcement of exercise by its effect on mood are all specific features that have been described for EA associated with eating disorders [36,37]. However, as EA may have high comorbidity and might also be associated with disorders other than eating disorders, it is likely that new specific features will be needed to define EA in relation to these additional disorders. This diversity of features essentially reflects the different ways in which EA can be understood and defined, and highlights the ongoing debate about the relationship between EA and other already recognized disorders.

1.4 The Relationship between Exercise Addiction and Other Mental Disorders

One key question that must be addressed before EA is recognized as a disorder is its relationship to other mental disorders. Underlying this question is the need to clarify whether EA can be considered a distinct disorder – that is, whether the problems associated with EA are due to the behaviour itself, or to other associated disorders [40,41]. It is essential to clarify this in order to enable future categorization of EA within the broader spectrum of mental disorders.

A key point in this debate is the distinction that Veale made between primary and secondary forms of EA [42]. EA is classified as primary when it represents a behavioural addiction in itself, whereas it is considered to be secondary when it co-occurs with another disorder, and according to the literature, secondary EA has generally been identified with an eating disorder, such as anorexia or bulimia nervosa [40,42]. In a primary addiction, the purpose of excessive exercise is to avoid something negative, although the affected individual may be unaware of this motivation. Here exercise provides a way to escape from a disturbing, persistent, and/or uncontrollable source of stress. However, in a secondary addiction, exercise is used as a means of achieving a goal that is characteristic of another dysfunction. For example, in individuals with anorexia nervosa, exercise may be used in addition to a strict diet as a means of losing weight.

The distinction between primary and secondary EA introduced by Veale has important clinical implications, as secondary EA would have a different aetiology to primary addiction, even though many symptoms of EA would be similar in both cases. The key feature suggested by Veale for distinguishing between the two forms of EA was that in primary addiction, exercise is the goal, whereas in secondary addiction, exercise is used to achieve another goal (e.g., weight loss), so exercise is only one of the possible means used to achieve this goal.

However, despite the clinical implications of this, there is currently no consensus on how to differentiate between primary and secondary EA. Although some authors assert that exercise may be a primary source of problems for some individuals [31], other authors maintain that primary EA has rarely been documented and is difficult to differentiate from problematic exercise associated with other disorders (e.g., eating disorders) [21,27,43,44]. Several factors may have contributed to the lack of agreement on how to recognize and differentiate between primary and secondary EA.

First, exercise has traditionally been seen as a healthy behaviour, so its harmful effects are often more likely to be recognized when they are associated with other disorders (e.g., eating disorders) than in relation to exercise itself [45]. Second, research has shown a relatively strong association between EA and eating disorders [46–49]. For example, Shroff et al. found that among a group of women who met the criteria for a diagnosis of anorexia and/or bulimia, 39% over-exercised, and this percentage rose to 54% in the subgroup of women with the purging subtype of anorexia nervosa [50]. Similarly, Klein et al. found that 48% of the women who were being treated for anorexia nervosa in their study were at risk of EA [51]. A recent systematic review and meta-analysis found that the effect size of the relationship between EA and eating disorders is larger in clinical populations [46], and it has been suggested that the risk of EA among individuals with eating disorders is more than 3.5-fold higher than that for individuals without an eating disorder [49].

Finally, a number of studies have understood the difference between primary and secondary addiction as being based on eating disorders alone [27,44,52,53]. These studies generally define primary EA in terms of the absence of an eating disorder. This view may have been influenced by the fact that Veale himself initially distinguished between primary and secondary dependence mainly with reference to the absence of an eating disorder. In 1987, he stated that 'A distinction should be made between primary exercise dependence and exercise dependence which is secondary to an eating disorder. A diagnostic hierarchy occurs in a case of exercise dependence, whereby the diagnosis of Anorexia Nervosa should be first excluded, followed by Bulimia Nervosa. A diagnosis of primary exercise dependence should only then be made' [42, p. 737].

However, a definition of EA based on the absence of eating disorders does not allow for the possibility that other disorders might be found to be associated with addiction to exercise. It is possible that secondary EA may be associated with other disorders as well as those related to eating. Subsequent research has indeed shown that eating disorders are only one type of disorder associated with EA. For example, in 1995, Veale established the operational diagnostic criteria for primary exercise dependence, and among them he highlighted the criterion that 'the preoccupation with exercise is not better accounted for by another mental disorder (e.g., as a means of losing weight or controlling calorie intake as in an eating disorder)' [40, p. 2]. Therefore Veale's distinction between primary and secondary EA appears to be more nuanced than the interpretation that has sometimes been conveyed in the literature.

To date, there has been little explicit recognition that a secondary form of EA may exist related to disorders other than eating disorders. For example, although Blaydon et al. defended the idea that EA is always secondary, they recognized that it may be linked either to a form of eating disorder or to excessive concern about body image [54]. In the same vein, McCabe and Vincent argued that exercise, together with dieting, is one of the most common ways of modifying body size and shape [39]. However, they understood that excessive exercise should be studied not only in relation to eating disorders, but also in relation to other disorders linked to modification of body size and shape. Exercise, together with control of nutrition, may be used to achieve specific body ideals (e.g., a muscular, thin, lean body) [55,56]. Research has indicated associations between EA and body dysmorphic disorder [57], and it has been suggested that muscle dysmorphia could be reclassified as an addiction to body image [58]. In addition, EA has been associated with other potential disorders related to body care and a concern about health, such as orthorexia nervosa [59,60]. Finally, some studies have found an association between behavioural addictions and other disorders, such as bipolar disorder [61,62]. Therefore classifications that establish a prevalence of primary addiction in individuals who do not present with a secondary exercise dependence associated with an eating disorder should be avoided, because they do not take into account the possibility that these individuals may have another associated mental disorder. This distinction has important practical and interventional implications, and should therefore be considered when defining what exactly authors consider to be EA.

1.5 Instruments for Assessing Exercise Addiction

To date, several self-report instruments have been designed to assess EA. In parallel with the evolution of the concept, the earliest instruments were one-dimensional assessments and generally referred to a specific activity. One of the first was the Commitment to Running Scale, in which EA was conceptualized as lying at one end of a continuum of exercise characterized by a strong commitment to running [63]. This scale was subsequently revised so that it could be applied to commitment to exercise more generally [64]. Other instruments that applied to running, such as the Obligatory Running Questionnaire [65], were based on the view that running addiction is a compulsive activity that shares psychological and behavioural symptoms with those seen in patients with anorexia nervosa. The Obligatory Running Questionnaire was later adapted so that it could be applied to exercise more generally, in the form of the Obligatory Exercise Questionnaire [66]. As the harmful consequences of exercise became more widely acknowledged, new scales such as the Running Addiction Scale [26] and the Negative Addiction Scale [67] were developed to assess both running addiction and general EA. However, these one-dimensional measures assessed only specific aspects of addiction, and did not provide a more comprehensive assessment of the construct [24].

Subsequently, multidimensional approaches have been developed that have drawn parallels between EA and substance addictions, and consequently defined EA as a varied set of symptoms [25,68]. For instance, Davis et al. developed the Commitment to Exercise Scale [69] after examining several published case studies of men and women with clear pathological or excessive exercise habits. The instrument has a two-factor, eight-item structure, and evaluates both the compulsive nature of exercise (e.g., feelings of guilt about missing a training session) and its pathological aspects (e.g., continuing to exercise despite illness or injuries).

Another early multidimensional instrument was the Exercise Dependence Questionnaire (EDQ), developed by Ogden et al. [70]. The authors based their conceptualization of problematic exercise on several criteria for substance dependence included in the DSM-IV, as well as on motivational factors (e.g., physical health, psychological health). Therefore, the EDQ conceptualizes EA as a combination of traditional elements of addiction (e.g., tolerance, withdrawal, repetitive behaviour), but also recognizes the psychosocial aspects of the problem (e.g., effects on interpersonal relationships). However, all of the measures that have been discussed so far lacked a cut-off criterion that could classify individuals at risk of addiction as symptomatic or asymptomatic.

According to recent reviews [71,72] the three most widely used instruments are the Exercise Dependence Scale (EDS) [24], the Exercise Addiction Inventory (EAI) [34], and the Compulsive Exercise Test (CET) [37]. These three instruments, unlike previous ones, have established cut-off points for classifying individuals at risk of exercise as symptomatic or asymptomatic. However, there are differences between these instruments with regard to the conceptualization of EA.

The EDS [24] defines EA in terms of the DSM-IV criteria for substance dependence [29]. This instrument has undergone a revision process [73], and its latest version contains a total of 21 items, comprising seven factors: (i) tolerance, (ii) withdrawal, (iii) intention effects, (iv) lack of control, (v) time, (vi) reduction in other activities, and (vii) continuance. Each of the subscales is represented by three items, and respondents are asked to indicate their response using a Likert scale ranging from 1 (never) to 6 (always). By operationalizing EA according to the seven criteria set out in the DSM-IV, the EDS provides information on the average of each of the factors or the average of the total score. Considering the first option, the EDS allows the differentiation of individuals into three groups, namely those who are at risk of addiction (i.e., with scores of 5–6 on the Likert scale for at least three of the seven criteria), those who are symptomatic (i.e., with scores of 3–4 on the Likert scale for at least three criteria, or scores of 5–6 combined with scores of 3–4 for three criteria, but without meeting the conditions for being at risk), and those who are asymptomatic (i.e., with scores of 1–2 on the Likert scale for at least three criteria, but without meeting the conditions for being symptomatic). The structure of the EDS has been validated in a number of different countries [74–77]. Although the EDS has a sound theoretical basis in that it utilizes the symptoms of dependence according to the criteria established in the DSM-IV, given the time it takes to administer the instrument and the complexity of the calculations necessary to identify individuals at risk of addiction, it is arguably not practicable for use in the daily work of sports doctors, physiotherapists, occupational therapists, and sports science professionals.

Unlike the EDS, the EAI [34,35] is an abbreviated and practical instrument for assessing the risk of EA. It operationalizes EA on the basis of the components of behavioural addictions [11,31–33], which is more in line with the new classification offered by the DSM-5. In the EAI, the symptoms of EA are operationalized through six components of behavioural addiction defined by Griffiths, namely salience, mood modification, tolerance, withdrawal symptoms, conflict, and relapse [33]. Each of the six items of the instrument reflects a component of addiction. In addition, based on the total score of its items, utilizing a five-point Likert scale, the EAI serves as a screening tool that can distinguish between individuals who are at risk of EA (i.e., scores of 24 or higher), have some symptoms (scores between 13 and 23), or have no symptoms of addiction (scores between 0 and 12). In a recent update of the EAI, a modification to the item response rating and a new cut-off point ($\geq$29) for identifying individuals at risk of EA were established [78].

Finally, the CET [37] is based on a cognitive–behavioural conceptualization of EA, viewing it primarily as a weight control behaviour that is maintained by concerns about body weight and body shape [36]. This instrument was specifically designed for use within the eating disorders domain. After the authors had examined the functioning of an initial pool of 31 items through three studies involving independent samples of women, they proposed a final model consisting of 24 items grouped into five factors: (i) avoidance and rule-driven behaviour; (ii) weight control exercise; (iii) mood improvement; (iv) lack of exercise enjoyment; and (v) exercise rigidity. Subsequent studies have reviewed the use of the instrument among different populations [36,79], including athletes [80]. Initially the authors did not propose cut-off points for the CET, but in a subsequent review of a sample of women with clinical eating disorders, Meyer et al. proposed a cut-off point (score of 15) to identify compulsive exercise among patients with eating disorders [79].

Although the EDS, EAI, and CET are currently the most commonly used psychometric instruments in EA research, the possibility cannot be ruled out that new instruments will be developed that will define EA according to criteria in newer editions of the clinical manuals (e.g., DSM-5), or in relation to other disorders as well as eating disorders. Moreover, with a few exceptions, such as the EAI [81], there is a lack of evidence for the instruments' validity and reliability, which would enable them to be used in different countries, cultures, and populations of people who exercise. This has made it difficult to compare the results of studies conducted in different settings and countries, including research in which a range of different instruments have been used to assess EA prevalence.

1.6 Prevalence of Exercise Addiction

The range of different criteria used to define EA, and the diversity of instruments used to assess it, have prevented an accurate estimate of its prevalence. A large number of studies indicate that the prevalence of EA is fairly low, ranging from 0.3% in the general population to 3% in populations who exercise regularly [22,33,73,82]. However, a few studies have reported EA prevalence rates of over 40% [44,83,84] – that is, five to ten times higher than the prevalence rates reported in most studies. The large discrepancy in EA prevalence may be related to three issues that have already been mentioned in this chapter.

First, there is no consensus on a precise conceptualization of the phenomenon. Therefore, as has been highlighted by Sicilia et al. [85], psychometric assessment tools are based on significant conceptual differences with regard to EA. For example, the early instruments, which use the term 'commitment' [63,64,69], conceptualize EA only as one end of the exercise continuum. However, as Szabo et al. have warned, the literature may include many studies of EA that measured excessive commitment to this behaviour but which did not assess negative consequences for the individual [86]. On the other hand, the fact that instruments with different conceptualizations assess different features of EA, can lead to differences between population groups. For instance, Weik and Hale assessed EA among people who exercised at a sports centre [87], using the Exercise Dependence Scale-Revised [73] and the

Exercise Dependence Questionnaire [70]. The results were interesting, indicating that when the EDS-R was used, men scored higher than women on abstinence, continuation, tolerance, lack of control, time, desired effects, and the total dependency value, whereas when the EDQ was used, women scored higher. These types of results show that the EDQ and the EDS-R assess different aspects of EA and classify either men or women as more addicted, depending on the instrument used and the dimension highlighted. Therefore it is logical to assume that instruments designed according to different conceptualizations of EA will show differences in the prevalence of EA [82], and systematic reviews that compare the prevalence of EA using instruments with different theoretical conceptualizations should take this fact into account.

Second, when a particular instrument has been modified or used differently, the reported prevalence is no longer informative. For example, Lejoyeux et al. reported an EA prevalence of 42% among a sample of fitness centre users [83]. However, as the authors themselves acknowledged, they had designed a specific scale for this study according to the diagnostic criteria of Hausenblas and Giacobbi [88], which may explain the discrepancy between their findings and the prevalence reported with other instruments, such as the EDS. Similarly, Serier et al. found an EA prevalence of 41.7% in a group of women with unequivocal body dissatisfaction [84]. However, although these authors assessed EA using the Obligatory Eating Questionnaire [66], for this study they arbitrarily created a cut-off point of above 50 to classify individuals as being at risk of EA. These practices may account for the significant discrepancy in the prevalence of EA even when it was assessed using the same instrument.

Third, the target populations in different studies of the prevalence of EA have varied widely, and have included, for example, runners, ultramarathoners, cyclists, university students, university student subgroups (e.g., sports science students), bodybuilders, fitness centre users, and elite athletes. Associated with this wide range of samples, not only sports modalities but also the amount of time spent exercising by participants in the studies have varied widely. Due to this great diversity, the items on the assessment instruments have been interpreted in different ways. For example, Szabo et al. suggest that the high scores on psychometric instruments that are shown by elite athletes compared with other populations should not be attributed to higher morbidity, but interpreted in relation to a high level of commitment to their profession [89]. Such differences in interpretation may well occur in relation to other population groups depending on, for example, gender or culture, and they highlight the need to provide evidence that instruments which are used to compare prevalence show measurement invariance across different population groups.

Finally, most studies of EA have been conducted using self-report assessment instruments. Consequently, the questionnaires and scales used have assessed the susceptibility to dysfunction in terms of the presence or intensity of symptoms associated with the addiction. These screening tools have limited diagnostic value, as a high score may not necessarily indicate harm or damage to the individual. If a person is identified as being at high risk for EA on the basis of psychometric instruments, this should be verified with a subsequent clinical interview and the use of scientifically validated criteria to confirm whether exercise behaviour has negative consequences for this individual. As has been highlighted by Szabo et al., there is a 'grey area' between the classification of being at risk and having a disorder, because the context of the individual and what exercise entails within that context is not known [89]. For the analysis of this context the clinical interview is a more precise approach than a self-report scale, especially with regard to assessment of the possible harm and lack of control that the behaviour produces in an individual.

1.7   Working towards a Consensus on the Definition of Exercise Addiction

Since the research conducted in the late 1970s, there has been a continuous attempt to identify the negative aspects of physical exercise as opposed to its more familiar positive effects. During that time, many terms associated with EA have emerged, such as 'exercise commitment', 'addictive exercise', 'abusive exercise', 'compulsive exercise', 'excessive exercise', 'exercise dependence', and 'obligatory exercise' [24,27,36,65,66,69]. These terms reflect the historical evolution of the phenomenon and the debates that have taken place around it [85]. Despite their conceptual diversity, all of these terms highlight possible negative effects of physical exercise, and describe a condition in which the practice of moderate or intense exercise becomes a disruptive behaviour for the individual. In an attempt to focus more on this common characteristic than on the differences, the terms 'problematic exercise' and 'morbid exercise' have been introduced [3,46,90]. These more generic terms refer to a form of exercise in which the individual loses control over their behaviour, and the behaviour is maintained despite the physical and psychological damage that it causes.

Despite the acceptance of the multidimensionality and complexity of EA, and the fact that this form of uncontrolled practice has negative consequences for the individual, the research findings have been somewhat ambiguous, due to the fact that to date the terminology of the constructs surrounding this phenomenon, their definition, and the measures designed to evaluate them have been so diverse. This presents a challenge for fundamental and applied research in the future, as the factors that prevail in, co-occur with, and perpetuate EA are still not entirely clear, making its prevention and treatment difficult.

1.8 Treatment of Exercise Addiction

Approaches to EA treatment often vary depending on whether the EA is viewed as primary or secondary. In cases of secondary addiction, treatment has been more frequent when EA has been associated with an eating disorder. Since eating disorders have long been recognized in the major diagnostic manuals (specifically the *Diagnostic and Statistical Manual of Mental Disorders*, and the *International Classification of Diseases*), there is much more literature available on how to treat them. However, there is also a risk that when EA and an eating disorder co-occur, the eating disorder will be treated at the expense of EA, as has been pointed out by Freitmuth et al. [68]. As eating disorders are the best known and officially recognized disorders, they may be the focus of treatment, and the problem of EA may remain hidden. Moreover, treatment for EA associated with other disorders and for primary EA is even more limited, since its prevalence is lower.

Since EA is not a recognized clinical disorder, one approach to looking for treatment strategies that may be effective has been to observe what specialists do in their daily practice. For example, Adams and Kirkby interviewed 24 sports physiotherapists to examine the problems they encountered and the strategies they used to treat patients with EA [91]. Re-education of the individual and especially their relationship with exercise can help to prevent the transformation of exercise activity from healthy to unhealthy. The authors highlighted the fact that many people who exercise are not aware that exercise is a problem [21,91], and consequently have difficulty recognizing and accepting a diagnosis of EA [45]. This inability to accept that exercise has become problematic reduces the likelihood of treatment success. Education programmes generally involve providing effective information and also details about training programmes to enable the individual to learn how to differentiate between unhealthy exercise-related behaviour and healthy behaviour. These education programmes are advisable when unhealthy behaviour (e.g., overtraining) appears to be the result of a poor understanding of the negative health consequences of the indivduals's actions [21]. However, in combination with re-education of exercisers, physiotherapists sometimes recommend alternative exercise activities, since by changing their exercise routine or alternating it with other types of exercise, people who exercise are sometimes able to modify their training schemes. One of the challenges for physiotherapists when implementing EA interventions is to differentiate between healthy and unhealthy exercise. Unlike other behaviours or substance intake, where engaging in the behaviour or consuming the substance do not bring any positive benefit, exercise is a type of behaviour that has proven health benefits when performed properly, and indeed is used as an adjunct for the treatment of other addictions and disorders, such as anxiety and stress disorders, schizophrenia, eating disorders, prenatal and postnatal depression, attention deficit hyperactivity disorder, and substance use disorders [1,7]. Research has shown that prolonged exercise withdrawal can have negative effects on mental health [1,92]. Therefore interventions should be focused not on the elimination of exercise behaviour, but on its control – that is, on re-education about its practice, where changing the activity or the way it is carried out can be an appropriate strategy.

Along with physiotherapists, other exercise-related professionals (e.g., trainers, instructors, personal trainers) may help to identify and attempt to prevent the negative consequences that exercise may have for some individuals. A survey by Colledge et al. showed that more than 70% of sports centre employees reported that they had observed at least one client whom they suspected of having an eating disorder or engaging in excessive exercise [93]. In addition, these employees reported that they felt able to identify when excessive exercise might be linked to eating disorders. This suggests that professionals who guide or supervise the daily exercise of population groups could (with the help of guideline documents or in collaboration with associations and centres for the treatment of these disorders) offer qualified guidance and/or educational programmes for the re-education of individuals with suspected EA.

However, in cases where a combination of educational programmes and the proposal of alternative forms of exercise is unsuccessful, physiotherapists and other professionals should direct the exerciser towards psychological treatment. For example, EA treatment can be based on treatments for other addictions, even though the processes involved in the different forms and manifestations of EA have not yet been fully clarified. Two interventions derived from the treatment of other addictions, namely motivational interviewing and cognitive–behavioural therapy, appear promising when applied to EA. Based on the transtheoretical model of motivation [94], motivational interviewing techniques aim to generate an intrinsic motivation for change. Individuals move from a pre-contemplative phase, in which there is not yet an intention to initiate treatment, to a phase that is more committed to action and behaviour change. This intervention is based on the view that an individual who is not at an appropriate stage to change is unlikely to commit to treatment. The second type of intervention, cognitive–behavioural therapy, is an effective form of therapy that has been used in substance abuse and other behavioural addictions, such as gambling disorder [95]. Here the therapist encourages the exercise addict to identify and correct the automatic and irrational thought processes that lead to emotions and maladaptive behaviours for that individual. In this way, the therapist helps them to understand how their irrational thinking can result in uncontrollable over-exercise. Cognitive–behavioural therapy can be combined with contingency management, in which the client is regularly tested to ensure that they do not engage in exercise in an undesirable way, so that their behaviour change is associated with rewards [21].

1.9 Future Directions in Exercise Addiction

In general, EA can be understood as a person's inner urge to exercise in an uncontrolled way, as they maintain the intention to exercise despite the harmful consequences of this behaviour [24,31,42]. However, EA is manifested in various forms, and can occur in individuals who exercise in different ways and for different reasons. Studies that examine features which are characteristic of individuals who regularly exercise may be informative. However, one limitation is that the lack of clinical criteria for defining EA makes it difficult to identify individuals as clinically addicted to exercise. This has led to the identification of features not only in other behavioural addictions and substance use disorders, but also in other disorders that might be associated with EA. However, the diagnosis and treatment of EA are still difficult to implement, due to the lack of specific diagnostic criteria for this particular addiction. Several points relating to the future development of these criteria should be considered.

First, the concept of EA has evolved over the past few decades, and a more satisfactory definition is needed that includes other associated terms and concepts. Although problematic exercise has been widely associated with eating disorders, there is increasing evidence that underlying some forms of EA there may also be other potential disorders associated with body image [58,59,96]. Therefore, the diversity of terms used to refer to problematic exercise may indicate that there are a number of different manifestations of EA. Therefore the development and validation of diagnostic criteria for EA will need to ensure that these are broad enough to capture the different features of all the possible manifestations of this disorder.

Second, although the multidimensional nature of EA is now well recognized, there is no consensus on the core criteria for this disorder. Furthermore, attempts to define addiction include different elements or dimensions that can occur separately depending not only on the type of addiction, but also on the personal characteristics and specific socio-cultural circumstances surrounding this behaviour. As a result, there has been a tendency to define this phenomenon as a set of elements when in fact each of those elements might represent different phenomena that do not usually occur together [12]. Some authors, such as Shaffer et al., have proposed alternative ways of thinking about this phenomenon, and suggested that addiction (which by definition could include EA) should be thought of as a syndrome that can have different forms of expression [97]. In this sense, a syndrome would allow EA to be thought of as a cluster of symptoms reflecting an abnormal underlying condition. Viewing EA as different clusters of symptoms would enable researchers in the field to explore this addiction as a broad family of different manifestations that can be individually distinguished by their specific combinations of factors, rather than as a single pathological phenomenon.

Finally, excessive exercising was conceptualized as a problem when the negative consequences of this behaviour for some individuals began to be investigated and assessed. If excessive exercise had no negative consequences, and the experience was always positive and beneficial in the ongoing development of the individual, it would not make sense to talk about addiction, at least in the sense in which this term is used to refer to other substances or behaviours [3,89,98]. Therefore, one future challenge will be to characterize the defining elements of EA. In this process, only elements that result in functional impairment, psychological distress, and/or a clear separation from normative behaviour in context should be considered [99]. This will require a more detailed examination of precisely when the individual's relationship to exercise behaviour becomes problematic. Similarly, although psychometric instruments can serve as a screening tool, context assessment is crucial when evaluating the harm that exercise causes in the individual's life [45,89].

References

1   Ashdown-Franks G, Firth J, Carney R et al. Exercise as medicine for mental and substance use disorders: a meta-review of the benefits for neuropsychiatric and cognitive outcomes. *Sports Med* 2020; 50: 151–70.

2   Davis C. Exercise abuse. *Int J Sport Psychol* 2000; 31: 278–89.

3   Szabo A, Demetrovics Z, Griffiths MD. Morbid exercise behavior: addiction or psychological escape? In: Budde H, Wegner M, eds. *The Exercise Effect on Mental Health: Neurobiological Mechanisms*. Routledge, 2018: 277–311.

4   Baekeland F. Exercise deprivation: sleep and psychological reactions. *Arch Gen Psychiatry* 1970; 22: 365–9.

5   Little JC. Athletic neurosis: a deprivation crisis. *Acta Psychiatr Scand* 1969; 45: 187–97.

6   Morgan WP. Negative addiction in runners. *Phys Sportsmed* 1979; 7: 56–70.

7   Fernandez DP, Kuss DJ, Griffiths MD. Short-term abstinence effects across potential behavioral addictions: a systematic review. *Clin Psychol Rev* 2020; 76: 101828.

8   American Psychiatric Association. *Diagnostic and Statistical Manual of Mental Disorders*, 5th ed. American Psychiatric Association, 2013.

9   World Health Organization. *ICD-11 for Mortality and Morbidity Statistics*. World Health Organization, 2019.

10 Grant JE, Potenza MN, Weinstein A, Gorelick DA. Introduction to behavioral addictions. *Am J Drug Alcohol Abuse* 2010; 36: 233–41.

11 Griffiths MD. Behavioural addiction: an issue for everybody? *Empl Couns Today* 1996; 8: 19–25.

12 Sussman S, Sussman AN. Considering the definition of addiction. *Int J Environ Res Public Health* 2011; 8: 4025–38.

13 Spada MM. Commentary on: are we overpathologizing everyday life? A tenable blueprint for behavioral addiction research. Problems with atheoretical and confirmatory research approaches in the study of behavioral addictions. *J Behav Addict* 2015; 4: 124–5.

14 Grant JE, Chamberlain SR. Expanding the definition of addiction: DSM-5 vs. ICD-11. *CNS Spectr* 2016; 21: 300–3.

15 Harvey J, Beamish R, Defrance J. Physical exercise policy and the welfare state: a framework for comparative analysis. *Int Rev Sociol Sport* 1993; 28: 53–64.

16 Plymire DC. Positive addiction: running and human potential in the 1970s. *J Sport Hist* 2004; 31: 297–315.

17 Maslow AH. *The Power of Self-Actualization*. Sounds True, 1992.

18 Kimiecik JC, Jackson SA. Optimal experience in sport: a flow perspective. In: Horn TS, ed. *Advances in Sport Psychology*. Human Kinetics, 2002: 501–27.

19 McInman AD, Grove JR. Peak moments in sport: a literature review. *Quest* 1991; 43: 333–51.

20 Glasser W. *Positive Addiction*. Harper & Row, 1976.

21 Adams J. Understanding exercise dependence. *J Contemp Psychother* 2009; 39: 231–40.

22 Allegre B, Souville M, Therme P, Griffiths MD. Definitions and measures of exercise dependence. *Addict Res Theory* 2006; 14: 631–46.

23 Estok PJ, Rudy EB. Physical, psychosocial, menstrual changes/risks, and addiction in the female marathon and nonmarathon runner. *Health Care Women Int* 1986; 7: 187–202.

24 Hausenblas HA, Symons-Downs D. How much is too much? The development and validation of the exercise dependence scale. *Psychol Health* 2002; 17: 387–404.

25 Hausenblas HA, Symons-Downs D. Exercise dependence: a systematic review. *Psychol Sport Exerc* 2002; 3: 89–123.

26 Chapman CL, De Castro JM. Running addiction: measurement and associated psychological characteristics. *J Sports Med Phys Fitness* 1990; 30: 283–90.

27 Bamber DJ, Cockerill IM, Rodgers S, Carroll D. Diagnostic criteria for exercise dependence in women. *Br J Sports Med* 2003; 37: 393–400.

28 Billieux J, Schimmenti A, Khazaal Y, Maurage P, Heeren A. Are we overpathologizing everyday life? A tenable blueprint for behavioral addiction research. *J Behav Addict* 2015; 4: 119–23.

29 American Psychiatric Association. *Diagnostic and Statistical Manual of Mental Disorders*, 4th ed. American Psychiatric Association, 2000.

30 Brown R. Some contributions of the study of gambling to the study of other addictions. In: Eadington WR, Cornelius JA, eds. *Gambling Behavior and Problem Gambling.* University of Nevada Press, 1993: 241–72.

31 Griffiths MD. Exercise addiction: a case study. *Addict Res* 1997; 5: 161–8.

32 Griffiths MD. The evolution of the 'components model of addiction' and the need for a confirmatory approach in conceptualizing behavioral addictions. *Düşünen Adam J Psychiatry Neurol Sci* 2019; 32: 179–84.

33 Griffiths MD. A 'components' model of addiction within a biopsychosocial framework. *J Subst Use* 2005; 10: 191–7.

34 Terry A, Szabo A, Griffiths MD. The Exercise Addiction Inventory: a new brief screening tool. *Addict Res Theory* 2004; 12: 489–99.

35 Griffiths MD, Szabo A, Terry A. The Exercise Addiction Inventory: a quick and easy screening tool for health practitioners. *Br J Sports Med* 2005; 39: e30.

36 Meyer C, Taranis L, Goodwin H, Haycraft E. Compulsive exercise and eating disorders. *Eur Eat Disord Rev* 2011; 19: 174–89.

37 Taranis L, Touyz S, Meyer C. Disordered eating and exercise: development and preliminary validation of the Compulsive Exercise Test (CET). *Eur Eat Disord Rev* 2011; 19: 256–68.

38 Yates A, Leehey K, Shisslak CM. Running—an analogue of anorexia? *N Engl J Med* 1983; 308: 251–5.

39 McCabe MP, Vincent MA. Development of body modification and excessive exercise scales for adolescents. *Assessment* 2002; 9: 131–41.

40 Veale D. Does primary exercise dependence really exist? In: Annett J, Cripps B, Steinberg H, eds. *Exercise Addiction: Motivation for Participation in Sport and Exercise: Proceedings of British Psychological Society, Division of Sport and Exercise Psychology.* British Psychological Society, 1995: 71–75.

41 Yates A, Leehey K, Shisslak CM. Running—an analogue of anorexia? *N Engl J Med* 1983; 308: 251–5.

42 Veale D. Exercise dependence. *Br J Addict* 1987; 82: 735–40.

43 Blaydon MJ, Lindner KJ, Kerr JH. Metamotivational characteristics of eating-disordered and exercise-dependent triathletes: an application of reversal theory. *Psychol Sport Exerc* 2002; 3: 223–36.

44 Blaydon MJ, Lindner KJ. Eating disorders and exercise dependence in triathletes. *Eat Disord* 2002; 10: 49–60.

45 Johnston O, Reilly J, Kremer J. Excessive exercise: from quantitative categorisation to a qualitative continuum approach. *Eur Eat Disord Rev* 2011; 19: 237–48.

46 Alcaraz-Ibáñez M, Paterna A, Sicilia A, Griffiths MD. Morbid exercise behaviour and eating disorders: a meta-analysis. *J Behav Addict* 2020; 9: 206–24.

47 Bamber DJ, Cockerill IM, Rodgers S, Carroll D. "It's exercise or nothing": a qualitative analysis of exercise dependence. *Br J Sports Med* 2000; 34: 423–30.

48 Cook B, Hausenblas HA. The role of exercise dependence for the relationship between exercise behavior and eating pathology: mediator or moderator? *J Health Psychol* 2008; 13: 495–502.

49 Trott M, Jackson SE, Firth J et al. A comparative meta-analysis of the prevalence of exercise addiction in adults with and without indicated eating disorders. *Eat Weight Disord* 2021; 26: 37–46.

50 Shroff H, Reba L, Thornton LM et al. Features associated with excessive exercise in women with eating disorders. *Int J Eat Disord* 2006; 39: 454–61.

51 Klein DA, Bennett AS, Schebendach J et al. Exercise 'addiction' in anorexia nervosa: model development and pilot data. *CNS Spectr* 2004; 9: 531–7.

52 Zmijewski CF. Howard MO. Exercise dependence and attitudes toward eating among young adults. *Eat Behav* 2003; 4: 181–95.

53 Maselli M, Gobbi E, Probst M, Carraro A. Prevalence of primary and secondary exercise dependence and its correlation with drive for thinness in practitioners of different sports and physical activities. *Int J Ment Health Addict* 2019; 17: 89–101.

54 Blaydon MJ, Lindner KJ, Kerr JH. Metamotivational characteristics of exercise dependence and eating disorders in highly active amateur sport participants. *Pers Individ Dif* 2004; 36: 1419–32.

55 Tod D, Edwards C. A meta-analysis of the drive for muscularity's relationships with exercise behaviour, disordered eating, supplement consumption, and exercise dependence. *Int Rev Sport Exerc Psychol* 2015; 8: 185–203.

56 Tod D, Edwards C, Hall G. Drive for leanness and health-related behavior within a social/cultural perspective. *Body Image* 2013; 10: 640–3.

57 Corazza O, Simonato P, Demetrovics Z et al. The emergence of exercise addiction, body dysmorphic disorder, and other image-related psychopathological correlates in fitness settings: a cross sectional study. *PLoS ONE* 2019; 14: e0213060.

58 Foster AC, Shorter GW, Griffiths MD. Muscle dysmorphia: could it be classified as an addiction to body image? *J Behav Addict* 2015; 4: 1–5.

59 Oberle CD, Watkins RS, Burkot AJ. Orthorexic eating behaviors related to exercise addiction and internal motivations in a sample of university students. *Eat Weight Disord* 2018; 23: 67–74.

60 Cena H, Barthels F, Cuzzolaro M et al. Definition and diagnostic criteria for orthorexia nervosa: a narrative review of the literature. *Eat Weight Disord* 2019; 24: 209–46.

61 Di Nicola M, Tedeschi D, Mazza M et al. Behavioural addictions in bipolar disorder patients: role of impulsivity and personality dimensions. *J Affect Disord* 2010; 125: 82–8.

62 Di Nicola M, Martinotti G, Mazza M et al. Quetiapine as add-on treatment for bipolar I disorder with comorbid compulsive buying and physical exercise addiction. *Prog Neuropsychopharmacol Biol Psychiatry* 2010; 34: 713–14.

63 Carmack MA, Martens R. Measuring commitment to running: a survey of runners' attitudes and mental states. *J Sport Psychol* 1979; 1: 25–42.

64 Corbin CB, Nielsen AB, Borsdorf LL, Laurie DR. Commitment to physical activity. *Int J Sport Psychol* 1987; 18: 215–22.

65 Blumenthal JA, Toole LCO, Jonathan L. Is running an analogue of anorexia nervosa? An empirical study of obligatory running and anorexia nervosa. *JAMA* 1984; 27: 520–3.

66 Pasman LN, Thompson JK. Body image and eating disturbance in obligatory runners, obligatory weightlifters, and sedentary individuals. *Int J Eat Disord* 1988; 7: 759–69.

67 Hailey BJ, Bailey LA. Negative addiction in runners: a quantitative approach. *J Sport Behav* 1982; 5: 150–4.

68 Freimuth M, Moniz S, Kim SR. Clarifying exercise addiction: differential diagnosis, co-occurring disorders, and phases of addiction. *Int J Environ Res Public Health* 2011; 8: 4069–81.

69 Davis C, Brewer H, Ratusny D. Behavioral frequency and psychological commitment: necessary concepts in the study of excessive exercising. *J Behav Med* 1993; 16: 611–28.

70 Ogden J, Veale D, Summers Z. The development and validation of the Exercise Dependence Questionnaire. *Addict Res* 1997; 5: 343–56.

71 Colledge F, Buchner U, Schmidt A, Walter M. Does exercise addiction exist? A brief review on current measurement tools and future directions. *Ment Health Addict Res* 2019; 4: 1–4.

72 Marques A, Peralta M, Sarmento H et al. Prevalence of risk for exercise dependence: a systematic review. *Sports Med* 2019; 49: 319–30.

73 Symons-Downs D, Hausenblas HA, Nigg CR. Factorial validity and psychometric examination of the Exercise Dependence Scale-Revised. *Meas Phys Educ Exerc Sci* 2004; 8: 183–201.

74 Lindwall M, Palmeira A. Factorial validity and invariance testing of the Exercise Dependence Scale-Revised in Swedish and Portuguese exercisers. *Meas Phys Educ Exerc Sci* 2009; 13: 166–79.

75 Sicilia A, González-Cutre D. Dependence and physical exercise: Spanish validation of the Exercise Dependence Scale-Revised (EDS-R). *Span J Psychol* 2011; 14: 421–31.

76 Müller A, Claes L, Smits D et al. Validation of the German version of the Exercise Dependence Scale. *Eur J Psychol Assess* 2013; 29: 213–19.

77 Costa S. Psychometric examination and factorial validity of the Exercise Dependence Scale-Revised in Italian exercisers. *J Behav Addict* 2012; 1: 186–90.

78 Szabo A, Pinto A, Griffiths MD, Kovácsik R, Demetrovics Z. The psychometric evaluation of the Revised Exercise Addiction Inventory: improved psychometric properties by changing item response rating. *J Behav Addict* 2019; 8: 157–61.

79 Meyer C, Plateau CR, Taranis L et al. The Compulsive Exercise Test: confirmatory factor analysis and links with eating psychopathology among women with clinical eating disorders. *J Eat Disord* 2016; 4: 1–9.

80 Plateau CR, Shanmugam V, Duckham RL et al. Use of the Compulsive Exercise Test with athletes: norms and links with eating psychopathology. *J Appl Sport Psychol* 2014; 26: 287–301.

81 Griffiths MD, Urbán R, Demetrovics Z et al. A cross-cultural re-evaluation of the Exercise Addiction Inventory (EAI) in five countries. *Sports Med Open* 2015; 1: 1–7.

82 Mónok K, Berczik K, Urbán R et al. Psychometric properties and concurrent validity of two exercise addiction measures: a population wide study. *Psychol Sport Exerc* 2012; 13: 739–46.

83 Lejoyeux M, Avril M, Richoux C, Embouazza H, Nivoli F. Prevalence of exercise dependence and other behavioral addictions among clients of a Parisian fitness room. *Compr Psychiatry* 2008; 49: 353–8.

84 Serier KN, Smith JE, Lash DN et al. Obligatory exercise and coping in treatment-seeking women with poor body image. *Eat Weight Disord* 2018; 23: 331–8.

85 Sicilia A, Paterna A, Alcaraz-Ibáñez M, Griffiths MD. Theoretical conceptualizations of problematic exercise in psychometric assessment instruments: a systematic review. *J Behav Addict* 2021; 10: 4–20.

86 Szabo A, Frenkl R, Caputo A. Relationship between addiction to running, commitment to running, and deprivation from running: a study on the Internet. In: *European Yearbook of Sport Psychology*, Vol. 1. European Federation of Sport Psychology, 1997: 130–47.

87 Weik M, Hale BD. Contrasting gender differences on two measures of exercise dependence. *Br J Sports Med* 2009; 43: 204–7.

88 Hausenblas HA, Giacobbi PR. Relationship between exercise dependence symptoms and personality. *Pers Individ Dif* 2004; 36: 1265–73.

89 Szabo A, Griffiths MD, de La Vega R, Mervó B, Demetrovics Z. Methodological and conceptual limitations in exercise addiction research. *Yale J Biol Med* 2015; 88: 303–8.

90 Chamberlain SR, Grant JE. Is problematic exercise really problematic? A dimensional approach. *CNS Spectr* 2020; 25: 64–70.

91 Adams J, Kirkby R. Exercise dependence: a problem for sports physiotherapists. *Aust J Physiother* 1997; 43: 53–8.

92 Weinstein AA, Koehmstedt C, Kop WJ. Mental health consequences of exercise withdrawal: a systematic review. *Gen Hosp Psychiatry* 2017; 49: 11–18.

93 Colledge F, Cody R, Pühse U, Gerber M. Responses of fitness center employees to cases of suspected eating disorders or excessive exercise. *J Eat Disord* 2020; 8: 1–9.

94 Prochaska JO, Redding CA, Evers KE. The transtheoretical model and stages of change. In: Glanz K, Rimer BK, Viswanath K, eds. *Health Behavior. Theory, Research, and Practice.* Jossey-Bass, 2015: 125–48.

95 Petry NM. *Pathological Gambling: Etiology, Comorbidity, and Treatment.* American Psychological Association, 2005.

96 Corazza O, Simonato P, Demetrovics Z et al. The emergence of exercise addiction, body dysmorphic disorder, and other image-related psychopathological correlates in fitness settings: a cross sectional study. *PLoS ONE* 2019; 14: 1–17.

97 Shaffer HJ, LaPlante DA, LaBrie RA et al. Toward a syndrome model of addiction: multiple expressions, common etiology. *Harv Rev Psychiatry* 2004; 12: 367–74.

98 Egorov AY, Szabo A. The exercise paradox: an interactional model for a clearer conceptualization of exercise addiction. *J Behav Addict* 2013; 2: 199–208.

99 Kardefelt-Winther D, Heeren A, Schimmenti A et al. How can we conceptualize behavioural addiction without pathologizing common behaviours? *Addiction* 2017; 112: 1709–15.

31.

32.

33.

34.

35.

36.

37.

38.

39.

Chapter

2

From Exercise to Addiction
The Fitspirational Era of Image and Performance Enhancement

Stefano Pallanti and Alice C. English

A triple ananke weighs upon us: the ananke of dogmas, the ananke of laws, the ananke of things. In *Notre-Dame de Paris* the author has denounced the first; in *Les Misérables* he has pointed out the second; in this book he indicates the third. With these three fatalities which envelop man is mingled the interior fatality, that supreme ananke, the human heart.
Victor Hugo

2.1 The Difference between Passion and Addiction

The term 'passion' derives from the Latin word 'passio', which is in turn derived from the word 'passus', the past participle of 'pati', meaning 'to suffer'. In Greek, however, the term πάθος (pathos) embodies the meaning of suffering but also indicates a strong emotion. Therefore the term 'passion' refers to a sense of suffering, pain, and an uncanny or strong feeling. Anyone can experience it – for example, some individuals may have a strong passion for music or sports. However, every passion contains hints of violence or love from one extreme to the other.

The term 'addiction' derives from the Latin word 'addictus', which was used in ancient Rome to describe a slave or servant who became enslaved because of unpaid debts, and whose condition lasted until the debt was paid off. In the scientific context, the term seemed appropriate for describing a person's slavery to a substance. Addiction is now defined as a condition in which a person, substance, or activity becomes necessary to meet our needs or make us feel better. In medicine, the term 'addiction' refers to a state in which an individual finds him- or herself in need of something, the withdrawal of which can cause a state of malaise.

Both terms – 'passion' and 'addiction' – allude to a strong, clamorous need. One of the features that distinguish passion from addiction is the subjective experience. Both subjective realities cause major emotional involvement, engaging one's full attention. However, the former is constructive whereas the latter is destructive. Passion corresponds to an intense flow of

25

emotional energy that leads to out-of-the-ordinary efforts, thus enabling one to overcome one's limits; conversely, dependence creates limits, paralyzing the will. Addiction is like an excess of passion. Both arise from the gratification derived from the experience – the more enjoyable and rewarding the engagement with the activity, the more likely it is that a bond will be created with it. Passionate individuals experience a strong attraction to the object of interest. Consider the example of a running enthusiast compared with an occasional runner. It is likely that the passionate runner will practise this activity every time they have an opportunity to do so, even in the most difficult weather conditions, and will invest more economic resources to buy the most suitable footwear and clothing, will consult books and magazines to improve their performance, and will experience positive emotions when engaging with running topics. Addiction produces an experience that is similar to passion, but with some important differences. An addicted runner will practise all of the behaviours implemented by the passionate runner, but will experience a condition of extreme malaise and uneasiness if prevented from engaging in this activity. The difference between passion and addiction lies in gratification. When the sensation of pleasure derived from the experience diminishes and there is a strong desire to experience again such positive emotions, passionate individuals may tend to increase the behaviours that previously produced gratification, thereby triggering a dependency mechanism.

Addiction is a condition in which free will – the ability to have control over one's actions – becomes obsolete. It is the addiction that has control, becoming the architect of one's actions, and compromising all aspects of one's life [1].

The *dualistic model of passion* proposes two types of passion, each of which is associated with particular outcomes and experiences [2]. 'Harmonious passion' is associated with an activity or object that one loves, accompanied by the internalization of one's identity, and is mostly associated with positive outcomes. In contrast, 'obsessive passion' is not under one's control (i.e., one is unable to control the urge to start or engage in the activity), is less adaptive, and is associated with negative outcomes.

Formal diagnosis of pathological addiction is usually based on the regular use of psychoactive substances (e.g., alcohol, tobacco, drugs such as heroin), but some behaviours can also be considered addictive, such as gambling, which is included in the fifth edition of the *Diagnostic and Statistical Manual of Mental Disorders (DSM-5)* [3], in the chapter on 'Substance-Related and Addictive Disorders', given the many phenotypic and genotypic similarities. In the DSM-5, the diagnosis of a substance use disorder is based on a pathological pattern of substance use behaviour. There are four main criteria: (i) the development of a substance-specific syndrome due to the recent ingestion of a substance; (ii) changes are attributable to the physiological effects of the substance on the central nervous system; (iii) the substance-specific syndrome causes clinically significant distress or impairment of important areas of functioning; (iv) the symptoms are not attributable to another medical condition and are not better explained by another mental disorder. Although many behavioural addictions can become problematic (e.g., shopping), to date only gambling has been officially included in the DSM-5, and the diagnostic criteria are similar to those for substance abuse, but without the requirement for actual ingestion of a substance.

2.2 Why Do People Exercise?

Exercise is a well-known and commonly used way to maintain physical health, but it is also beneficial for many aspects of mental health. We can exercise to lose weight, build muscular mass, have a reason to get out and socialize at the gym, change some aspect of our body shape, or improve many aspects of our psychological well-being. Regular physical exercise has been shown to be correlated with improvements in memory, self-esteem, mood, motivation, sleep, and chronic pain [4], and is beneficial for patients who are at high cardiovascular risk [5]. People may use exercise to relax and to reduce anxiety, and it has been shown to be effective in relieving symptoms of stress and anxiety-related disorders [6]. Regularly practising yoga could be just as effective in improving physical and mental health among both healthy and diseased populations, due to the down-regulation of the hypothalamic–pituitary–adrenal axis and the sympathetic nervous system [7]. Some studies have demonstrated its benefits for patients with major depression [8], and research suggests that regular moderate-intensity exercise reduces the inflammation that may be associated with depression symptoms [9] and could serve as an effective form of preventive care [10]. Physical exercise has been shown to be beneficial for hippocampal neurogenesis [11], and it has been indicated as a prospective treatment for preventing the cognitive decline that is typical of many disorders, such as Alzheimer's disease. The antidepressant effect of exercise is believed to be linked to its effect on the hippocampus [12].

2.3 The Relationship of Body Image and Body Dissatisfaction to Exercise and Eating Behaviour

Nowadays the concept of *body image* – that is, how a person perceives their own body and how beautiful or attractive they feel – has an important role in the individual's physical and psychological well-being. We pay so much attention to how we look in certain clothes, to our skin and hair, and above all to how our body looks that we are constantly seeking new ways to improve our body image. Every year there is a new diet, a new exercise to get rid of stomach fat, clothing that is specifically designed to sculpt the body in a certain way, make-up routines that can potentially alter facial characteristics, and the list goes on and on. Social media have an important effect on body image, due to the constant posting of photos or videos of illusionary beauty and perfection, and there is ample proof of the effects of social networking sites on body image and eating behaviours [13]. One study found that exposure to photos that promoted thin ideals led to higher levels of body dissatisfaction among a population of young female students [14]. The social media boom has also led to an increase in eating disorders among the female population, even if at the onset of such disorders there is a complex interaction between sociocultural and genetic factors [15] and many aspects of body image, body concerns, and body dissatisfaction [16].

Body dissatisfaction is a negative attitude towards one's body, due to a perceived discrepancy between one's actual appearance and the ideal body image that one has in terms of weight or physical form. This can have negative psychological and physical consequences. It is at the root of the development of non-adaptive behaviours such as abuse of plastic surgery, and excessive exercise has been shown to be one of the major risk factors for the development of eating disorders [17]. One study has found a clear correlation between body dissatisfaction, exercise addiction (EA), and eating disorders [18], highlighting the fact that body dissatisfaction leads to a higher level of exercise addiction, especially in the female population.

In Europe, eating disorders affect an alarming number of individuals, and psychological and physical complications are a cause for concern. Among women, anorexia nervosa is reported in 1–4% of the population, bulimia in 1–2%, and binge eating in 1–4%. In contrast, among men the prevalence of eating disorders is much lower, at around 0.3–0.7% [19]. Worldwide, the estimated prevalence of eating disorders is around 8.4% for women, compared with 2.2% for men, with a higher prevalence in the USA [20].

Both anorexia nervosa and bulimia are characterized by an intense fear of gaining weight, and the behaviours that individuals with these disorders adopt are aimed at preventing weight gain. Affected individuals also have a severely distorted perception of their body weight and body shape, and weight is severely overestimated in the case of anorexia nervosa. Commonly observed negative behaviours among individuals with eating disorders include excessive exercise and motor restlessness. These are well-documented characteristics of anorexia nervosa, especially in association with high levels of anxiety and somatization [21]. It has been reported that a tendency to engage in excessive exercise is generally associated with a lower body mass index, younger age groups, perfectionism, and the purging subtype of anorexia [22]. One study has found that excessive exercise occurs during the acute phase of the disorder, and that premorbid levels of activity are an important predictor of future behaviour [23].

In an attempt to explain the finding of excessive exercise among individuals with anorexia nervosa, Rizk et al. have proposed an interesting and comprehensive model that takes into account a whole range of factors, including the individual's personal history, their interactions with their environment, and the pathological consequences [24]. The model is divided into five periods. Period 0 consists of the factors that preceded the disorder, such as childhood activity levels, participation in weight-oriented sports, and having a more physically active parent. Period 1 is characterized by the onset of the disorder, with an increase in physical exercise to achieve weight loss being associated with an early age of onset of the disorder. In Period 2, physical exercise becomes a coping strategy to alleviate psychological distress, suppress negative feelings and stress, and relieve the main symptoms of the disorder, such as feelings of body dissatisfaction and the drive for thinness. Once exercise has been established as a coping mechanism, there is an increased need to engage in physical activity, when even normal daily activities are transformed into a way to exercise more (e.g., walking for long distances instead of driving). Period 3 is the acute phase, in which physical activity has a compulsive component that is no longer under the individual's control. There is still also a voluntary component, driven by factors such as body dissatisfaction and preoccupation with avoiding weight gain. Period 4 consists of the long-term effects, which are not yet well established, as weight-recovered patients still have a tendency to engage in excessive exercise, and also have a higher tendency to drop out of treatment programmes [25]. Compulsiveness is not uncommon in individuals with anorexia nervosa or other eating disorders, and it has been reported that patients with anorexia nervosa who were identified as high-level exercisers tended to be significantly more likely to exhibit obsessive-compulsive personality traits [26]. Another study found the same association with both obsessive-compulsive personality traits and obsessive-compulsive symptomatology [27]. This overlap may be due not only to the psychopathological similarities but also to a shared underlying neurobiological dysfunction.

A Delphi study has suggested that, in cases of anorexia nervosa, 'compulsive exercise' is the preferred term for describing the unhealthy exercise behaviour that is observed in adolescents with this disorder [28]. In this context, Dittemer et al. have proposed several specific diagnostic criteria for defining compulsive exercise in cases of anorexia [29]. First, the exercise is performed according to rigid rules or in response to an obsession that causes significant distress. The objective of the exercise is to alleviate distress or prevent negative consequences. Second, the exercise behaviour is time-consuming (more than 1 hour a day) and interferes with the individual's daily activities, impairs other areas of their life, or may even be continued despite injury or lack of enjoyment. Finally, the individual must have insight into the negative effect that the exercise is having on their life, and its excessive nature. The authors also identify three subtypes of compulsive exercise that can be seen in individuals with anorexia nervosa, namely vigorous exercise, a marked increase in daily movement, and motor restlessness [29]. However, the Delphi study showed three major differences in terms of the proposed criteria once a consensus had been reached for the term 'compulsive exercise' [28]. Dittemer et al. found that compulsive exercise is predominantly motivated by the fear of weight gain and by dissatisfaction with body shape, and is not related to thoughts about caloric intake [29]. In addition, they pointed out that many people may exercise in secret, which may affect the reliability of assessments. Finally, the amount of time spent thinking about exercise was considered to be important. Patients with eating disorders tend to devote a great deal of time to food-related thoughts and preoccupations, so the focus on the amount of time spent thinking about exercise was considered to be misleading.

Nonetheless, body image and its perception have a major impact on both eating behaviour and exercise behaviour, and athletes in particular are a population that warrant close study. An Icelandic research group studied 755 elite athletes representing 20 different sports, and found that at least 17.9% of them showed moderate or severe body image dissatisfaction, and 18.2% were above the clinical cut-off for concern about body image [30]. This study also confirmed previous findings of a higher prevalence of body image issues in women. However, disorders in male athletes should not be underestimated, given the fact that disordered eating behaviour and body dissatisfaction have been reported in 27% of athletes [31]. When defining excessive exercise or addiction to exercise in this population, the matter becomes more complicated. Most assessment tools ask about the amount of time spent engaging in exercise behaviour, and as exercise is athletes' main occupation there is clearly a need for some specific adaptations for this category. De la Vega et al. found an association between obsessive passion and addiction to exercise in athletes, although these findings may need to be revised to take into account the differences between professional and non-competitive athletes [32].

2.4 Neurobiology of Movement and Exercise

Movement involves a large number of areas of the motor system in the brain, including the primary motor cortex, premotor cortex, cerebellum, dorsolateral prefrontal cortex, basal ganglia, and cingulate, among others. These interact and coordinate with external signals, using auditory or visual cues that activate the sensory-specific areas and the limbic system. However, the precise sequence of events, and the many processes involved between conscious thought and actually executing a movement, are not yet understood. In the context of movement it is worth mentioning that free will is a problematic subject. We generally believe that we choose whether to make a movement – the perception that we have free will – and this makes us think that we are entirely responsible for the movements that we make. A movement takes place when the motor cortex is activated and sends a movement command [33], gathering signals from the rest of the brain. Therefore movement really begins at a subconscious level, guided by internal and external cues, starting from the mesial areas, whereas volition involves other areas in the parietal lobe and insular cortex [34]. When a movement plan is guided by an internal cue, such as decisional processes or matters of voluntary choice, activation occurs in different areas to those activated by external cues, such as a sensory input. Internal cues activate areas such as the dorsolateral prefrontal cortex, the supramarginal gyrus, and the ipsilateral posterior parietotemporal regions, which indicates that these areas are involved in selection of a movement. External cues activate different areas, starting with the bilateral supplementary motor cortex and the presupplementary motor cortex, which indicates a possible role in stimulus–response mapping [35].

Intention and planning are two important yet distinct processes, and actualization of the movement requires coordination between many different areas, including the supplementary motor area, which if damaged can result in problems with complex activities such as bimanual coordination, as has been demonstrated in monkeys [36].

From a neurobiological perspective, exercise involves the dopaminergic reward system, which is also associated with most addictions. Thus the involvement of this system could explain the similarity to other behavioural addictions, which are characterized by well-known symptoms such as abstinence, withdrawal, craving, and tolerance. Studies of patients with Parkinson's disease (PD) have shown promise in confirming that there is a link between the dopaminergic system and physical exercise. PD is one of the most frequent neurodegenerative movement disorders, and the loss of dopaminergic neurons in the pars compacta of the substantia nigra leads to its development [37]. A study that used positron emission tomography (PET) and functional magnetic resonance imaging (fMRI) to monitor dopamine release in response to aerobic exercise in individuals with PD found increased activity of the ventral striatum in anticipation of a 75% probability of reward, and increased dopamine release in the caudate nucleus [38]. These changes are probably due to the mesolimbic dopaminergic pathway, and suggest that exercise is beneficial for corticocortical plasticity and dopamine release. Exercise training is now often combined with pharmaceutical treatments, such as levodopa, to increase dopamine release and improve the plasticity of the cortical striatum [39].

At this point it is worth mentioning the phenomenon of 'runner's high'. After an intense long-distance run, some individuals experience a sense of euphoria, which is probably correlated with opioid binding in the prefrontal and orbitofrontal cortices, the anterior cingulate cortex, bilateral insula, parainsular cortex, and temporoparietal regions [40]. Aerobic exercise has been linked to changes in the anterior cingulate cortex, which is essential for mood regulation, resulting in an increase in volume of this region [41]. In adolescents, aerobic exercise programmes have been shown to increase levels of brain-derived neurotrophic factor (BDNF), which is essential for neuroplasticity and cognitive activity [42]. In the elderly, group dancing activities induce a similar increase in BDNF levels, as well as volume increases in the cingulate cortex, insula, corpus callosum, and sensorimotor cortex, improving both cognitive and attentional functioning [43].

The relationship between sound and movement has recently been studied. When people exercise, they usually use some form of auditory stimulus, and can synchronize their movements with such stimuli, using mechanisms in different cortical areas, the basal ganglia, and the cerebellum [44]. Music and other rhythmic sounds also serve as a useful distraction during exercise (e.g., from fatigue, pain, or external factors), and have been demonstrated to be effective in prolonging and improving exercise performance [45].

2.5 Brief Neurobiology of Addiction

Behavioural addiction is a relatively new topic, with many studies focusing on the underlying neurobiological mechanisms in an attempt to understand the causes of the repetitive and harmful behaviours. There are many similarities with substance abuse.

Most of the research data are based on animal models, which are not always good predictors of human responses. However, substances and certain behaviours both have a clear effect on the reward system. Koob and Volkov have discussed a series of studies that debate the role of such a system and the neuroadaptations that occur in cases of addiction, and they identify three separate phases of addiction, namely intoxication, withdrawal, and finally craving and relapse [46]. They postulate that five main circuits, which are engaged in succession, contribute to the onset of addiction: (i) the mesolimbic dopamine system; (ii) the ventral striatum; (iii) the ventral striatum/dorsal striatum/thalamus circuits; (iv) the dorsolateral frontal cortex/inferior frontal cortex/hippocampus circuits; and (v) the amygdala [46]. With regard to abuse of substances (e.g., cocaine), the first neuroadaptation involves changes in glutamate activity within the mesolimbic dopamine system. Subsequently, the activation of dopamine lead to activation of the ventral striatum, with a reduction in glutamatergic activity during the withdrawal stage, and increased glutamatergic activity during cue-induced substance seeking. The role of the ventral striatal thalamic system is to translate to the dorsal striatum, setting in train the automatic and habitual behaviour that is often observed in substance abuse. When the behaviour becomes addictive, there is loss of functionality of the frontal cortex, which results in deficits in executive control functions. This in turn causes the lack of good decision making that results in the individual's perception of the salience of drugs or substances rather than natural stimuli. Behavioural addictions involve many related areas similar to those just described, such as deficits in the frontal cortex and the striatum [47].

However, genetic and environmental factors may also play a role in the development of addiction, and some studies have found volumetric and structural differences in individuals with behavioural addictions.

2.6 Exercise as an Addiction

Negative exercise behaviour has been observed and described in the practice of a number of different sports, such as running [48] and bodybuilding [49], and these studies depict a clinical picture very similar to that seen in substance abuse cases. Griffiths reported one of the very first clinical case studies [50]. The case concerned a 25-year-old woman, who to a large extent prioritized exercising over everything else in her life, was constantly thinking about her next training session, and would spend at least 6 hours a day on exercise-related matters. This pattern had developed over a period of 5 years, from only participating in evening classes initially to an all-consuming activity. If the woman was interrupted while exercising, her mood would change dramatically, and she would become irritable or agitated. Even when she had an injury she would still find a way to continue exercising. Her excessive exercising had repercussions for her finances, education, and personal life, and she was unable to stop the excessive exercising for more than a few days because she constantly 'felt an urge' to engage in this behaviour. This particular case includes all the components of addiction, namely salience, tolerance, withdrawal, euphoria, conflict, loss of control, and relapse.

EA could be viewed as part of the cluster of behavioural addictions, along with gambling. However, the individual's characteristics also need to be considered. Therefore differential diagnosis is a crucial aspect of the evaluation, which should consider possible comorbidities (e.g., eating disorders, body dysmorphia), and the many features that such addiction can share with other psychopathologies (e.g., obsessive-compulsive disorder). Many studies have found high rates of co-occurring disorders in people who are vulnerable to EA, such as mood and anxiety-related disorders, substance abuse or other addictive behaviours, and borderline personality disorder [51]. As we shall discuss later on, many conceptualized models have attempted to explain the development of EA. Some studies have suggested that body dissatisfaction is a likely underlying cause [52], whereas others have proposed the involvement of neuroticism as a trait, with overactivation of the reward system accompanied by underactivation of the inhibitory system, as the mechanism underlying EA [53]. One of the main components of any addiction is loss of control, which is also present or at risk of development in people with EA. In cases of addiction, loss of control refers to the inability to stop or regulate the behaviour, to resist the behaviour, or to choose from a wide range of behaviours [54].

In an attempt to gain a better understanding of the neurobiological basis of the development of behavioural addictions, Brand et al. have proposed another interesting model, namely the Interaction of Person-Affect-Cognition-Execution (I-PACE) model [55]. They argue that addictive behaviours develop as a result of interactions between predisposition, cognitive and affective responses, the perception of internal or external triggers, and executive functions. When impaired executive functions, such as inhibitory control, are associated with cue reactivity and craving, this could potentially lead to the development of addictive behaviours. Brand et al. also suggest that an imbalance between the ventral striatum, the amygdala, and the dorsolateral prefrontal areas may be involved in the early stages of the addiction process, whereas imbalances in the dorsal striatum are involved in the later stage (i.e., there is a transition of processing from the ventral to the dorsal striatum). This connectivity has been studied in individuals with internet gaming disorder [56]. It was found that observed activity in the ventral striatum was negatively correlated with cue-induced craving, whereas activation in the dorsal striatum was positively correlated with the duration of the addictive disorder.

Recently, the National Institute of Mental Health established the Research Domain Criteria (RDoC) project, which was designed to facilitate research on mental disorders by attempting to overcome the limitations of the dimensional approaches, focusing on specific factors such as genetics, environment and, most importantly, neurobiology [57]. The RDoC describes five domains: Negative Valence Systems; Positive Valence Systems; Cognitive Systems; Social Processes; and Arousal and Regulatory Systems (see Figure 2.1). A sixth domain, Sensorimotor Systems, has recently been added, which is responsible for motor behaviour, its control and implementation, and the future perfection of movements over time. In the case of behavioural addictions, such as gambling disorder, the main domains involved are the Positive Valence Systems and the Cognitive Systems [58]. The former is responsible for behaviours such as reward-seeking or consummatory behaviour, whereas the latter is the route of cognitive processes, such as cognitive control and response inhibition. We could hypothesize that the same systems are at least to some extent involved in EA. However, a consensus on its definition has yet to be reached.

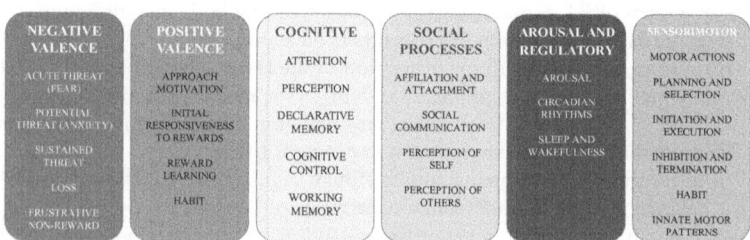

Figure 2.1 Research Domain Criteria (RDoC) system.

A study using the Delphi technique [59], which is mainly applied in health sciences when the available knowledge is uncertain or incomplete [60], attempted to determine the features of EA by consulting individuals with relevant expertise. These participants defined different characteristics of people who exercise excessively, such as negative perfectionism (when a pathological behaviour is largely maintained by negative reinforcement) and obsessive-compulsive drive (when the person is unable to give up the behaviour or the craving, and experiences loss of enjoyment of the behaviour itself). In addition, a hedonic component was described (the anticipation of the reward, and the minimization of the negative outcomes and the effects of withdrawal).

As with most addictive behaviours, onset of EA tends to occur during adolescence, and to be associated with a higher prevalence of mental distress. One study has reported a prevalence of EA of 4% among school athletes [61]. However, other studies have found more variable prevalence values, ranging from 3% among people who exercise regularly [62] to 8.6% among runners [63]. In addition, during the COVID-19 pandemic the restrictions imposed during the various lockdowns influenced people's exercising habits. Although the requirement to stay at home decreased exercise volume, a 15.2% risk of EA was found within a population of exercisers from Spanish-speaking nations [64]. These estimates are usually obtained using two instruments, such as the Exercise Dependence Scale (EDS) [65] and the Exercise Addiction Inventory (EAI) [66], which both contain items relating to the DSM-IV criteria for addictions. However, the estimates obtained using these tools do not provide a precise prevalence figure, given the nature of this addiction, but rather they identify individuals who are more at risk or who are symptomatic. The target population must also be considered when using such questionnaires, as there are significant differences in responses between occasional or leisure exercisers and professional exercisers or those who exercise for a living.

2.7 Conceptual Models of the Development of Exercise Addiction

Reflecting the difficulties in defining EA and delineating a cut-off between problematic and non-problematic exercise, many different conceptual models of its development have been proposed.

The first such model, presented by Thompson and Blanton, was based on the physiological adaptations of organisms to exercise that could result in addiction [67]. They suggested that exercise may lead to an adaptive decrease in energy, with a reduction in sympathetic output, as a result of which the individual needs to engage in higher levels of activity in order to achieve the desired level of arousal and avoid feeling lethargic. However, these effects are limited, so the individual may have to increase the amount of exercise needed over time (i.e., they develop tolerance).

Szabo proposed a different approach, which takes into account the effect of exercise on life stress [68]. We have already discussed how some individuals may use exercise as a way to cope with stress and anxiety. Once exercise has been established as a coping mechanism, the person tends to depend on the behaviour on a daily basis, believing it to be healthy and adaptive. However, this behaviour may start to interfere with various aspects of their life, such as work and social responsibilities, and if they do not exercise they lose a coping mechanism.

Freimuth et al. proposed four phases which lead to the development of exercise addiction [69]. In the first phase the individual finds exercise pleasurable and regards it as a leisure activity. During the second phase they notice the benefits of exercise, become aware of its positive effect on their mood and appearance, and therefore are inclined to exercise more. In the third phase the addiction, as described by Szabo [68], becomes a major coping mechanism, and exaggerated exercising has negative consequences for both physical and mental health. The fourth stage exhibits all the typical characteristics of a fully developed addiction, such as tolerance, withdrawal symptoms, impact on mood, and relapse.

However, as Egorov and Szabo have pointed out [70], these models do not explain why exercise in particular is chosen as a coping mechanism. These authors propose a conceptual model based on a 'black box', which represents a large pool of personal and situational factors that are unique to the individual. This hypothetical black box can only be 'opened' after a formal diagnosis has been made, and it pinpoints all of the possible factors that could help to determine the motivation behind the exercise behaviour. Thus this model considers many environmental and situational determinants as the primary motive for choosing exercise behaviour, and these motives are mainly related to improving health and/or preventing illness (e.g., preventing weight gain). However, the most important component of this model relates to the appearance of a suddenly emerging reaction to a stressor that causes psychological distress over which the individual has no control. The presence of a stressor in this model underlines the fact that EA has a rapid onset (rather than a slow progression), characterized by the sudden loss of control, which creates an instant need to find a coping mechanism. The choice of mechanism will be determined by the person's unique combination of individual factors, situational factors, and antecedents of exercise behaviour.

2.8 Treatment Proposals

To date, few treatments have been proposed for EA. Cognitive–behavioural therapy may be a valid approach, although evidence in support of its effectiveness is scarce [71]. Any treatment plan should consider all of the individual factors involved, and the assessment must determine whether the addiction is primary in nature (in which case it will cause the individual more distress), or whether it is secondary to another disorder (most commonly an eating disorder). Weinstein and Weinstein suggest that the first step in treating these patients should involve focusing on motivation, helping the patient to understand the long-term effects of the behaviour, and motivating them to proceed with treatment [71]. Once their agreement to treatment has been obtained, the next step involves identifying the thoughts underlying the EA, correcting them, and adopting alternative behavioural strategies. Given that exercise is fundamentally a healthy habit, complete abstinence is not recommended, and the best approach would be to aim to reach a point where the person can still exercise in moderation.

However, there are many valid treatment options for other behavioural addictions. As with most addictions, three steps are involved in treating such disorders, namely detoxification, recovery, and relapse prevention [72]. Detoxification is a very delicate and fundamentally important stage, which results in abstinence from the behaviour, accompanied by possible withdrawal symptoms. Recovery consists of the individual's ability to learn new behaviours aimed at controlling craving and developing motivation to avoid falling back into the negative habits. The final stage of treatment is a long-term plan to prevent relapse.

With regard to pharmacological treatments, many options are available, such as opioid-receptor antagonists, antidepressants, antipsychotics, and glutamate-receptor antagonists. The most commonly used approach is a calibrated combination of pharmacological treatment and some other option, such as cognitive–behavioural therapy. Naltrexone, which is known to be an efficient drug for the treatment of substance abuse, has also shown efficacy in the treatment of behavioural addictions such as kleptomania, trichotillomania, and impulsive-compulsive disorders [73]. In addition, naltrexone has been shown to be very effective in the treatment of gambling disorder [74]. There are many treatment options for gambling disorder, due to the extensive body of research on its underlying neurobiological mechanisms. For this behavioural addiction, opioid-receptor antagonists appear to be one of the best treatment options, and lithium or other mood stabilizers have shown efficacy in cases of comorbidity with bipolar disorder [75]. Selective serotonin reuptake inhibitors (SSRIs), such as fluvoxamine, have been reported to be effective in reducing the symptoms of gambling disorder in the presence of co-occurring disorders, such as anxiety or depression [76]. Glutamatergic pharmacotherapies are of interest because it has been postulated that a glutamatergic imbalance is responsible for reward-seeking behaviour, and one study has demonstrated reasonable efficacy of topiramate for the treatment of gambling disorder [77]. Bupropion has been proposed as a pharmaceutical treatment for patients with internet video game addiction, and it has been found that after 6 weeks of sustained-release bupropion treatment, both cravings and brain activity in the dorsolateral prefrontal cortex were reduced [78]. This drug has also shown greater efficacy than escitalopram in reducing impulsive behaviour and attentional difficulties in the treatment of patients with internet gaming disorders with co-occurring major depression [79]. Citalopram has been successfully used for the treatment of sex addiction [80]. Han et al. conducted another study in which methylphenidate, a stimulant that is usually administered to patients with attention deficit hyperactivity disorder (ADHD), was administered to 62 children with internet video game addiction [81]. In this trial they observed a significant decrease in both internet video game addiction and overall internet use, combined with a reduction in ADHD symptoms. Finally, it has been suggested that valproate and other anti-epileptic drugs could be beneficial for the treatment of internet addiction [82].

With regard to psychological interventions, again there are many options available, and they focus on all steps of addiction treatment, including withdrawal, craving management, relapse prevention, improvement of impulsive behaviour, and emotion regulation.

Cognitive–behavioural therapy (CBT) is one of the most widely used therapies, and has been demonstrated to be effective in the treatment of a wide range of psychological disorders, including substance use disorders [83] and other behavioural addictions. The focus of this intervention is on the maladaptive cognitions or schemas that maintain problematic behaviours and cause significant distress for the individual. The objective of CBT is to identify such cognitions and behaviours, to challenge them through cognitive restructuring, and to propose alternatives to replace the negative patterns, thereby alleviating the emotional distress. Relapse prevention strategies are a fundamental element of treatment. A relapse consists of a setback that occurs during the treatment process, where the individual reverts to engaging in the targeted behaviour [84]. It is very important for the patient to learn how to identify possible triggers so that they can increase their ability to cope with these potential situations. CBT has shown promising beneficial effects in the treatment of gambling disorders, with one study reporting that this therapeutic approach significantly improved the symptoms of gambling disorders, and that these improvements were maintained at a 12-month follow-up [85]. For patients with internet addiction, CBT may be the treatment of choice. One study found that patients were able to manage their symptoms successfully by the eighth session of treatment, and these improvements were found to have been maintained up to 6 months later [86].

Self-help and online-based therapies have been proposed for the treatment of addictions, and have been demonstrated to be both effective and low-cost interventions [87]. With regard to behavioural addictions, one study found that self-help treatment reduced the symptoms of gambling disorder and improved both perceived self-efficacy and life satisfaction, even over the long term [88]. Oei et al. reported that a self-help cognitive–behavioural treatment programme for problem gamblers produced a significant improvement in symptoms, gambling cognitions, gambling urges, and correlated psychological states [89]. There is a 12-step programme for gambling disorders (similar to that for alcohol addiction) which could be combined with individual therapy to potentially achieve a higher level of engagement with therapy and a lower rate of relapse [90].

Mindfulness-based interventions, which have been of particular interest in recent years, have been used in the treatment of a wide spectrum of disorders, and adopted specifically for relapse prevention. The practice of mindfulness has been embedded within Western psychology, where awareness, non-judgement, and acceptance are the fulcrum, and the focus is on managing day-to-day experiences and distress. This approach is commonly used, for example, in the treatment of anxiety disorders that focus on rumination and worry [91]. A recent review has found that the use of mindfulness-based interventions that are aimed at emotion regulation is effective for both behavioural and substance addictions [92]. The most commonly used therapy was mindfulness-based relapse prevention, and the probability of recovery was increased when this was combined with other active treatments.

Transcranial magnetic stimulation (TMS) is a safe, non-invasive, and cost-effective way to study cortical excitability via magnetic stimulation [93]. Repetitive transcranial magnetic stimulation (rTMS) is a type of TMS in which electricity is used to generate a magnetic field that is applied to various areas of the brain. Depending on the intensity and frequency of the magnetic field, this results in the creation of magnetic impulses that induce depolarization and current flow in neurons such that, when there is continuous stimulation over time, permanent changes in plasticity can be produced. To date it has been successfully used in the treatment of many disorders; for example, it can be used to treat depression by stimulating the prefrontal area daily for 4–6 weeks [94]. In patients with addictions, the application of rTMS to stimulate the dorsolateral cortex can be used to modify the circuits that are responsible for the cognitive processes involved in addiction and craving [95]. Zack et al. studied how rTMS can cause a significant decrease in cravings and better cognitive functioning in a small sample of patients with gambling disorders [96]. They found that high-frequency rTMS and continuous theta burst stimulation (cTBS) can mitigate gambling reinforcement and behaviour. Gay et al. reported that a single session of rTMS applied over the left dorsolateral prefrontal cortex showed significant success in reducing cue-induced craving [97]. A more recent study of the application of rTMS to the left dorsolateral prefrontal cortex in a group of 8 patients with gambling disorder lasted for several weeks [98]. The first phase of the study involved preliminary screening of all the patients. This was followed by a 2-week intensive rTMS treatment phase (generally twice a day for 5 days a week, although some sessions occurred twice a day for 1 day a week). The final phase was a follow-up to assess whether the effects were maintained after 3 months. The researchers found a mean reduction of 71.2% in the scores on the assessment scale used, and a significant decrease in the number of days spent on gambling behaviour; all of these improvements were maintained during the follow-up period. The use of cTBS to stimulate the pre-supplementary motor area (pre-SMA) could be effective in enhancing cognitive control and response inhibition. More detailed research involving a controlled double-blind study will be needed to clarify this.

Transcranial direct current stimulation (tDCS) is another non-invasive brain stimulation treatment that has been implemented in the treatment of addictions. This methodology modulates brain activity by passing electric current through electrodes that are placed on the scalp. This allows the modification of membrane potential and neuron activity, which over the long term can diminish or enhance certain functions. When applied to the dorsolateral prefrontal cortex, tDCS can have an effect on craving and impulse control in individuals with gambling disorder. One study has demonstrated that stimulation twice a day for 10 days, followed by two 3-month follow-up maintenance periods in which sessions only take place once a week or every 2 weeks, can reduce both craving and impulse control [99]. The same results were obtained in subsequent studies, in which stimulation of the dorsolateral prefrontal cortex by tDCS was found to improve decision making and cognitive abilities [100]. In this population, stimulation of the right dorsolateral prefrontal cortex was able to reduce craving [101].

2.9 Conclusion

This chapter began with a discussion of the difference between passion and addiction, then considered some of the reasons why people may exercise, and then went on to examine the common features that are shared by neurobiology of addiction and of exercise. The characteristics of EA were then described with reference to a series of conceptual models that have been proposed to explain the phenomenon. Finally, several possible treatments that are more commonly used for other behavioural addictions were suggested as potentially being suitable for use in EA.

Distinguishing between passion and addiction in relation to behaviours is not an easy task. The novelty of our approach lies in avoiding the tendency to only consider subjective or intersubjective characteristics when we should in fact be adopting an ecological approach. Such an approach enables us to start to understand not only the subjective nature of the determinants of these behaviours, but also how many other external factors, of which we are unaware, act as triggers. According to the quantum theory of consciousness it is not possible to distinguish between passion and addiction, as there is such a large overlap between the two, and such a view is consistent with the redefinition of substance use in the DSM-5, including the removal of the term 'abuse' [3]. There is a continuum that extends from a small use or repetition to great psychological distress for the individual. We need to alert the population to this, because this phenomenon is encouraged by our present-day environment, and particularly by the 'cyber environment'.

Shoshana Zuboff has promoted the concept of 'surveillance capitalism' [102]. This is the idea that we live in a world in which there is a constant need or craving to extract information and data – a need that has been instigated by the Internet and that leads to the development of a series of behaviours which can become compulsive, guided by feelings of anxiety and restlessness. We live in an era in which any passion, including exercise, can become exaggerated, and we feel under pressure to practise some kind of activity that will build our self-esteem. The 'cyber environment' is specifically designed to uncover our desires and passions, which act on our ventral striatum, and by a series of individually designed reinforcements to compel us to behave in certain ways. For example, if we search once on the Internet for athletic equipment, we will then be repeatedly encouraged to do so in the future. The role of the environment needs to be highlighted and further investigated, especially with regard to how some environments can now be considered to be obesogenic – that is, they lead to obesity in individuals or entire populations by promoting sedentary behaviour and/or high food intake [103]. These types of environments can be a major cause of compulsive behaviours, which include not only eating behaviour but behaviours in general. Addiction and compulsiveness are inevitable in humans, and indeed all mammals, given the innate brain mechanisms that promote excess consumption even when there is no immediate requirement for this, in order to cope with future periods of deprivation. For example, some animals in hot arid regions consume excessive amounts of water in order to increase the likelihood of their survival.

When we want to evaluate something, we cannot consider it in isolation, because it is just one mechanism within a whole system. Democritus (c. 460–c. 370 BCE) claimed that all of reality was composed of tiny particles, or atoms, which move constantly. These atoms, he maintained, are indivisible and in constant movement, which leads them to either attach to each other or become increasingly distant from each other, resulting in the creation of matter, which then undergoes transformation and dies. Democritus suggested that the difference between one object and another lies in the difference between the atoms – their shape, their dimension, and their disposition when they join together. He also distinguished between objective and subjective qualities, thus creating a form of dualism. He proposed that objective characteristics are determined by the formation of atoms, whereas subjective characteristics are determined by the interpretation or perception of atoms, and therefore are not real. The problem with this theory of dualism is that in practice there cannot be such a radical distinction between the two. It is necessary to go beyond the I-PACE model proposed by Brand et al. [55]. Not only do we need to consider the internal and external triggers that may or may not be perceived (the cue reactivity/craving and reduced inhibitory control associated with the development of addictions), but also we should specifically be broadening our knowledge of the environment's role, especially in the present era of constant cyber activity.

We should be shaping the environments in which we live so as to promote a balanced way of life, as well as focusing more on prevention strategies and interventions for all populations, and endeavouring to understand better how they interact with their environment. In parallel with this we need to become more aware of our behaviours and our subjective vulnerabilities, while keeping control over our actions and the person we may want to become.

References

1   Wegner DM. *The Illusion of Conscious Will*. MIT Press, 2002.

2   Vallerand RJ. On the psychology of passion: in search of what makes people's lives most worth living. *Can Psychol* 2008, 49: 1–13.

3   American Psychiatric Association. *Diagnostic and Statistical Manual of Mental Disorders*, 5th ed. American Psychiatric Association, 2013.

4   Archer T, Josefsson T, Lindwall M. Effects of physical exercise on depressive symptoms and biomarkers in depression. *CNS Neurol Disord Drug Targets* 2014; 13: 1640–53.

5   Sharman JE, La Gerche A, Coombes JS. Exercise and cardiovascular risk in patients with hypertension. *Am J Hypertens* 2015; 28: 147–58.

6   Kandola A, Stubbs B. Exercise and anxiety. *Adv Exp Med Biol* 2020; 1228: 345–52.

7   Ross A, Thomas S. The health benefits of yoga and exercise: a review of comparison studies. *J Altern Complement Med* 2010; 16: 3–12.

8   Ströhle A. Physical activity, exercise, depression, and anxiety disorders. *J Neural Transm (Vienna)* 2009; 116: 777–84.

9   Paolucci EM, Loukov D, Bowdish DME, Heisz JJ. Exercise reduces depression and inflammation but intensity matters. *Biol Psychol* 2018; 133: 79–84.

10   Strawbridge WJ, Deleger S, Roberts RE, Kaplan GA. Physical activity reduces the risk of subsequent depression for older adults. *Am J Epidemiol* 2002; 156: 328–34.

11   Ma CL, Ma XT, Wang JJ et al. Physical exercise induces hippocampal neurogenesis and prevents cognitive decline. *Behav Brain Res* 2017; 317: 332–9.

12   Bjørnebekk A, Mathé AA, Brené S. The antidepressant effect of running is associated with increased hippocampal cell proliferation. *Int J Neuropsychopharmacol* 2005; 8: 357–68.

13 Holland G, Tiggemann M. A systematic review of the impact of the use of social networking sites on body image and disordered eating outcomes. *Body Image* 2016; 17: 100–10.

14 Tiggemann M, Hayden S, Brown Z, Veldhuis J. The effect of Instagram "likes" on women's social comparison and body dissatisfaction. *Body Image* 2018; 26: 90–7.

15 Polivy J, Herman CP. Causes of eating disorders. *Annu Rev Psychol* 2002; 53: 187–213.

16 Aparicio-Martinez P, Perea-Moreno AJ, Martinez-Jimenez MP et al. Social media, thin-ideal, body dissatisfaction and disordered eating attitudes: an exploratory analysis. *Int J Environ Res Public Health* 2019; 16: 4177.

17 McLean SA, Paxton SJ. Body image in the context of eating disorders. *Psychiatr Clin North Am* 2019; 42: 145–56.

18 Freire GLM, da Silva Paulo JR, da Silva AA et al. Body dissatisfaction, addiction to exercise, and risk behaviour for eating disorders among exercise practitioners. *J Eat Disord* 2020; 8: 23.

19 Keski-Rahkonen A, Mustelin L. Epidemiology of eating disorders in Europe: prevalence, incidence, comorbidity, course, consequences, and risk factors. *Curr Opin Psychiatry* 2016; 29: 340–5.

20 Galmiche M, Déchelotte P, Lambert G, Tavolacci MP. Prevalence of eating disorders over the 2000–2018 period: a systematic literature review. *Am J Clin Nutr* 2019; 109: 1402–13.

21 Peñas-Lledó E, Vaz Leal FJ, Waller G. Excessive exercise in anorexia nervosa and bulimia nervosa: relation to eating characteristics and general psychopathology. *Int J Eat Disord* 2002; 31: 370–5.

22 Shroff H, Reba L, Thornton LM et al. Features associated with excessive exercise in women with eating disorders. *Int J Eat Disord* 2006; 39: 454–61.

23 Davis C, Katzman DK, Kaptein S et al. The prevalence of high-level exercise in the eating disorders: etiological implications. *Compr Psychiatry* 1997; 38: 321–6.

24 Rizk M, Mattar L, Kern L et al. Physical activity in eating disorders: a systematic review. *Nutrients* 2020; 12: 183.

25 El Ghoch M, Calugi S, Pellegrini M et al. Measured physical activity in anorexia nervosa: features and treatment outcome. *Int J Eat Disord* 2013; 46: 709–12.

26 Davis C, Kaptein S, Kaplan AS, Olmsted MP, Woodside DB. Obsessionality in anorexia nervosa: the moderating influence of exercise. *Psychosom Med* 1998; 60: 192–7.

27 Davis C, Kaptein S. Anorexia nervosa with excessive exercise: a phenotype with close links to obsessive-compulsive disorder. *Psychiatry Res* 2006; 142: 209–17.

28 Noetel M, Dawson L, Hay P, Touyz S. The assessment and treatment of unhealthy exercise in adolescents with anorexia nervosa: a Delphi study to synthesize clinical knowledge. *Int J Eat Disord* 2017; 50: 378–88.

29 Dittmer N, Jacobi C, Voderholzer U. Compulsive exercise in eating disorders: proposal for a definition and a clinical assessment. *J Eat Disord* 2018; 6: Article 42.

30 Kristjánsdóttir H, Sigurðardóttir P, Jónsdóttir S, Þorsteinsdóttir G, Saavedra J. Body image concern and eating disorder symptoms among elite Icelandic athletes. *Int J Environ Res Public Health* 2019; 16: 2728.

31 Goltz FR, Stenzel LM, Schneider CD. Disordered eating behaviors and body image in male athletes. *Braz J Psychiatry* 2013; 35: 237–42.

32 de la Vega R, Parastatidou IS, Ruíz-Barquín R, Szabo A. Exercise addiction in athletes and leisure exercisers: the moderating role of passion. *J Behav Addict* 2016; 5: 325–31.

33 Hallett M. Physiology of free will. *Ann Neurol* 2016; 80: 5–12.

34 Hallett M. Volitional control of movement: the physiology of free will. *Clin Neurophysiol* 2007; 118: 1179–92.

35 Ariani G, Wurm MF, Lingnau A. Decoding internally and externally driven movement plans. *J Neurosci* 2015; 35: 14160–71.

36 Yip DW, Lui F. *Physiology, Motor Cortical.* StatPearls Publishing, 2021.

37 Balestrino R, Schapira AHV. Parkinson disease. *Eur J Neurol* 2020; 27: 27–42.

38 Sacheli MA, Neva JL, Lakhani B et al. Exercise increases caudate dopamine release and ventral striatal activation in Parkinson's disease. *Mov Disord* 2019; 34: 1891–900.

39 Feng YS, Yang SD, Tan ZX et al. The benefits and mechanisms of exercise training for Parkinson's disease. *Life Sci* 2020; 245: 117345.

40 Boecker H, Sprenger T, Spilker ME et al. The runner's high: opioidergic mechanisms in the human brain. *Cereb Cortex* 2008; 18: 2523–31.

41 Lin K, Stubbs B, Zou W et al. Aerobic exercise impacts the anterior cingulate cortex in adolescents with subthreshold mood syndromes: a randomized controlled trial study. *Transl Psychiatry* 2020; 10: 155.

42 Azevedo KPM, de Oliveira VH, Medeiros GCBS et al. The effects of exercise on BDNF levels in adolescents: a systematic review with meta-analysis. *Int J Environ Res Public Health* 2020; 17: 6056.

43 Rehfeld K, Lüders A, Hökelmann A et al. Dance training is superior to repetitive physical exercise in inducing brain plasticity in the elderly. *PLoS ONE* 2018; 13: e 0196636.

44 Damm L, Varoqui D, De Cock VC, Dalla Bella S, Bardy B. Why do we move to the beat? A multi-scale approach, from physical principles to brain dynamics. *Neurosci Biobehav Rev* 2020; 112: 553–84.

45 Bood RJ, Nijssen M, van der Kamp J, Roerdink M. The power of auditory-motor synchronization in sports: enhancing running performance by coupling cadence with the right beats. *PLoS ONE* 2013; 8: e70758.

46 Koob G, Volkow N. Neurocircuitry of addiction. *Neuropsychopharmacology* 2010; 35: 217–38.

47 Leeman RF, Potenza MN. A targeted review of the neurobiology and genetics of behavioural addictions: an emerging area of research. *Can J Psychiatry* 2013; 58: 260–73.

48 Morgan WP. Negative addiction in runners. *Phys Sportsmed* 1979; 7: 55–77.

49 Hurst R, Hale B, Smith D, Collins D. Exercise dependence, social physique anxiety, and social support in experienced and inexperienced bodybuilders and weightlifters. *Br J Sports Med* 2000; 34: 431–5.

50 Griffiths MD. Exercise addiction: a case study. *Addict Res* 1997; 5: 161–8.

51 Colledge F, Sattler I, Schilling H et al. Mental disorders in individuals at risk for exercise addiction–a systematic review. *Addict Behav Rep* 2020; 12: 100314.

52 Alcaraz-Ibáñez M, Paterna A, Sicilia Á, Griffiths MD. A systematic review and meta-analysis on the relationship between body dissatisfaction and morbid exercise behaviour. *Int J Environ Res Public Health* 2021; 18: 585.

53 Huang Q, Huang J, Chen Y et al. Overactivation of the reward system and deficient inhibition in exercise addiction. *Med Sci Sports Exerc* 2019; 51: 1918–27.

54 Griffiths MD. Is "loss of control" always a consequence of addiction? *Front Psychiatry* 2013; 4: 36.

55 Brand M, Wegmann E, Stark R et al. The Interaction of Person-Affect-Cognition-Execution (I-PACE) model for addictive behaviors: update, generalization to addictive behaviors beyond internet-use disorders, and specification of the process character of addictive behaviors. *Neurosci Biobehav Rev* 2019; 104: 1–10.

56 Liu L, Yip SW, Zhang JT et al. Activation of the ventral and dorsal striatum during cue reactivity in Internet gaming disorder. *Addict Biol* 2017; 22: 791–801.

57 Insel TR. The NIMH Research Domain Criteria (RDoC) Project: precision medicine for psychiatry. *Am J Psychiatry* 2014; 171: 395–7.

58 Marras A, Makris N. A Research Domain Criteria (RDoC) approach to Gambling Disorder: focus on preference-based decision-making and response inhibition. *Arch Behav Addict* 2019; 1. DOI: https://doi.org/10.30435/ABA.01.2019.06.

59 Macfarlane L, Owens G, Cruz Bdel P. Identifying the features of an exercise addiction: a Delphi study. *J Behav Addict* 2016; 5: 474–84.

60 Niederberger M, Spranger J. Delphi technique in health sciences: a map. *Front Public Health* 2020; 8: 457.

61 Lichtenstein MB, Griffiths MD, Hemmingsen SD, Støving RK. Exercise addiction in adolescents and emerging adults – validation of a youth version of the Exercise Addiction Inventory. *J Behav Addict* 2018; 7: 117–25.

62 Márquez S, de la Vega R. La adicción al ejercicio: un trastorno emergente de la conducta [Exercise addiction: an emergent behavioral disorder.] *Nutr Hosp* 2015; 31: 2384–91.

63 Lukács A, Sasvári P, Varga B, Mayer K. Exercise addiction and its related factors in amateur runners. *J Behav Addict* 2019; 8: 343–9.

64 de la Vega R, Almendros LJ, Barquín RR et al. Exercise addiction during the COVID-19 pandemic: an international study confirming the need for considering passion and perfectionism. *Int J Ment Health Addict* 2022; 20: 1159–70.

65 Hausenblas HA, Downs DS. How much is too much? The development and validation of the Exercise Dependence Scale. *Psychol Health* 2002; 17: 387–404.

66 Terry A, Szabo A, Griffiths M. The Exercise Addiction Inventory: a new brief screening tool. *Addict Res Theory* 2004; 12: 489–99.

67 Thompson JK, Blanton P. Energy conservation and exercise dependence: a sympathetic arousal hypothesis. *Med Sci Sports Exerc* 1987; 19: 91–9.

68 Szabo A. The impact of exercise deprivation on well-being of habitual exercises. *Aust J Sci Med Sport* 1995; 27: 68–75.

69 Freimuth M, Moniz S, Kim SR. Clarifying exercise addiction: differential diagnosis, co-occurring disorders, and phases of addiction. *Int J Environ Res Public Health* 2011; 8: 4069–81.

70 Egorov AY, Szabo A. The exercise paradox: an interactional model for a clearer conceptualization of exercise addiction. *J Behav Addict* 2013; 2: 199–208.

71 Weinstein A, Weinstein Y. Exercise addiction – diagnosis, bio-psychological mechanisms and treatment issues. *Curr Pharm Des* 2014; 20: 4062–9.

72 Potenza MN, Sofuoglu M, Carroll KM, Rounsaville BJ. Neuroscience of behavioral and pharmacological treatments for addictions. *Neuron* 2011; 69: 695–712.

73 Mouaffak F, Leite C, Hamzaoui S et al. Naltrexone in the treatment of broadly defined behavioral addictions: a review and meta-analysis of randomized controlled trials. *Eur Addict Res* 2017; 23: 204–10.

74 Kim SW, Grant JE, Adson DE, Shin YC. Double-blind naltrexone and placebo comparison study in the treatment of pathological gambling. *Biol Psychiatry* 2001; 49: 914–21.

75 Yip SW, Potenza MN. Treatment of gambling disorders. *Curr Treat Options Psychiatry* 2014; 1: 189–203.

76 Hollander E, DeCaria CM, Mari E et al. Short-term single-blind fluvoxamine treatment of pathological gambling. *Am J Psychiatry* 1998; 155: 1781–3.

77 Berlin HA, Braun A, Simeon D et al. A double-blind, placebo-controlled trial of topiramate for pathological gambling. *World J Biol Psychiatry* 2013; 14: 121–8.

78 Han DH, Hwang JW, Renshaw PF. Bupropion sustained release treatment decreases craving for video games and cue-induced brain activity in patients with Internet video game addiction. *Exp Clin Psychopharmacol* 2010; 18: 297–304.

79 Nam B, Bae S, Kim SM, Hong JS, Han DH. Comparing the effects of bupropion and escitalopram on excessive internet game play in patients with major depressive disorder. *Clin Psychopharmacol Neurosci* 2017; 15: 361–8.

80 Wainberg ML, Muench F, Morgenstern J et al. A double-blind study of citalopram versus placebo in the treatment of compulsive sexual behaviors in gay and bisexual men. *J Clin Psychiatry* 2006; 67: 1968–73.

81 Han DH, Lee YS, Na C et al. The effect of methylphenidate on Internet video game play in children with attention-deficit/hyperactivity disorder. *Compr Psychiatry* 2009; 50: 251–6.

82 Przepiorka AM, Blachnio A, Miziak B, Czuczwar SJ. Clinical approaches to treatment of Internet addiction. *Pharmacol Rep* 2014; 66: 187–91.

83 McHugh RK, Hearon BA, Otto MW. Cognitive behavioral therapy for substance use disorders. *Psychiatr Clin North Am* 2010; 33: 511–25.

84 Hendershot CS, Witkiewitz K, George WH, Marlatt GA. Relapse prevention for addictive behaviors. *Subst Abuse Treat Prev Policy* 2011; 6: 17.

85 Petry NM, Ammerman Y, Bohl J et al. Cognitive-behavioral therapy for pathological gamblers. *J Consult Clin Psychol* 2006; 74: 555–67.

86 Young KS. Cognitive behavior therapy with Internet addicts: treatment outcomes and implications. *Cyberpsychol Behav* 2007; 10: 671–9.

87 Newman MG, Szkodny LE, Llera SJ, Przeworski A. A review of technology-assisted self-help and minimal contact therapies for drug and alcohol abuse and smoking addiction: is human contact necessary for therapeutic efficacy? *Clin Psychol Rev* 2011; 31: 178–86.

88 Boudreault C, Giroux I, Jacques C et al. Efficacy of a self-help treatment for at-risk and pathological gamblers. *J Gambl Stud* 2018; 34: 561–80.

89 Oei TPS, Raylu N, Lai WW. Effectiveness of a self help cognitive behavioural treatment program for problem gamblers: a randomised controlled trial. *J Gambl Stud* 2018; 34: 581–95.

90 Petry NM. Gamblers Anonymous and cognitive–behavioral therapies for pathological gamblers. *J Gambl Stud* 2005; 21: 27–33.

91 Rodrigues MF, Nardi AE, Levitan M. Mindfulness in mood and anxiety disorders: a review of the literature. *Trends Psychiatry Psychother* 2017; 39: 207–15.

92 Sancho M, De Gracia M, Rodríguez RC et al. Mindfulness-based interventions for the treatment of substance and behavioral addictions: a systematic review. *Front Psychiatry* 2018; 9: 95.

93 Duan X, Yao G, Liu Z, Cui R, Yang W. Mechanisms of transcranial magnetic stimulation treating on post-stroke depression. *Front Hum Neurosci* 2018; 12: 215.

94 Rizvi S, Khan AM. Use of transcranial magnetic stimulation for depression. *Cureus* 2019; 11: e4736.

95 Gorelick DA, Zangen A, George MS. Transcranial magnetic stimulation in the treatment of substance addiction. *Ann N Y Acad Sci* 2014; 1327: 79–93.

96 Zack M, Cho SS, Parlee J et al. Effects of high frequency repeated transcranial magnetic stimulation and continuous theta burst stimulation on gambling

reinforcement, delay discounting, and Stroop interference in men with pathological gambling. *Brain Stimul* 2016; 9: 867–75.

97 Gay A, Boutet C, Sigaud T et al. A single session of repetitive transcranial magnetic stimulation of the prefrontal cortex reduces cue-induced craving in patients with gambling disorder. *Eur Psychiatry* 2017; 41: 68–74.

98 Pettorruso M, Martinotti G, Montemitro C et al. Multiple sessions of high-frequency repetitive transcranial magnetic stimulation as a potential treatment for gambling addiction: a 3-month, feasibility study. *Eur Addict Res* 2020; 26: 52–6.

99 Martinotti G, Chillemi E, Lupi M et al. Gambling disorder and bilateral transcranial direct current stimulation: a case report. *J Behav Addict* 2018; 7: 834–7.

100 Soyata AZ, Aksu S, Woods AJ et al. Effect of transcranial direct current stimulation on decision making and cognitive flexibility in gambling disorder. *Eur Arch Psychiatry Clin Neurosci* 2019; 269: 275–84.

101 Martinotti G, Lupi M, Montemitro C et al. Transcranial direct current stimulation reduces craving in substance use disorders: a double-blind, placebo-controlled study. *J ECT* 2019; 35: 207–11.

102 Zuboff S. *The Age of Surveillance Capitalism.* Profile Books, 2019.

103 Lake A, Townshend T. Obesogenic environments: exploring the built and food environments. *J R Soc Promot Health* 2006; 126: 262–7.

From Exercise to Addiction: An Introduction to the Phenomenon

The COVID-19 Pandemic

A Novel Risk Factor for Exercise Addiction and Related Disorders

Franca Ceci, Francesco Di Carlo, Julius Burkauskas, Giovanni Martinotti, and Massimo di Giannantonio

3.1 Exercise Addiction: Definition, Epidemiology, and Aetiopathogenesis

Regular exercise can be defined as a set of complex, planned, structured, and repetitive movement activities that are performed with sufficient frequency, intensity, and duration to be effective in promoting health and preventing disease in individuals of all ages [1–3].

In addition to its beneficial effects, physical activity can also be associated with impaired mental health, being associated with problems such as excessive exercising and overtraining syndrome [2]. In 1979, William Morgan discussed studies which had shown that exaggerated exercise could lead both to physical injury and to the neglect of daily responsibilities such as those related to work and family. He suggested that, in these extreme cases, exercise could represent a new type of addiction, associated with withdrawal symptoms, problems in daily functioning, exercising despite medical contraindications to this, and harmful effects on social relationships and work [4]. Subsequently the term 'exercise addiction' began to be used [5–7].

Hausenblas and Symons Downs characterized exercise addiction (EA) on the basis of criteria that are modifications of the criteria for substance dependence listed in the text revision of the fourth edition of the *Diagnostic and Statistical Manual of Mental Disorders (DSM-IV-TR)* [8–10]. EA is not officially included in any of the international classifications of mental disorders. However, based on its main symptoms, it could potentially be classified within the category of behavioural addictions [5,11–13].

EA can be either a primary disorder or secondary to another disorder, most commonly an eating disorder such as anorexia nervosa or bulimia [14–16].

The epidemiological distribution of EA is very heterogeneous. There are two possible reasons for this – first, the psychometric tools used in the assessment, and second, the target population studied.

Several scales have been developed for the assessment of EA, but none of them have been validated in a clinical population, and the samples studied were often of small size or belonged to specific risk categories (e.g., members of fitness clubs, professional athletes). Published studies have reported prevalence estimates ranging from 3.2% to 52% [15,17–20]. This high variability can be partly explained by Schipfer and Stoll's Exercise-Addiction/Exercise-Commitment Model (EACOM), which suggests that the degree of passion and perfectionism could have a moderating effect on EA [21].

The screening tools currently used for EA measure an individual's susceptibility to developing this condition. This susceptibility is often incorrectly assessed in terms of the number of hours of physical activity or the level of commitment to it, sometimes confusing passion or being a professional athlete with the actual disorder [17]. To establish a true diagnosis, an individual psychiatric evaluation is necessary, which is difficult to apply on a large scale [17].

The two most popular screening tools, the Exercise Dependence Scale (EDS) [8,9] and the Exercise Addiction Inventory (EAI) [22], both give an estimated prevalence of EA of around 3% among individuals who regularly engage in physical activity [23–27]. With regard to the general population, rigorous and methodologically valid prevalence studies of EA are lacking. However, some observational studies have reported a prevalence ranging from 0.3% to 0.5% [26,27], whereas a meta-analysis gave a prevalence estimate of 3%.

The EDS conceptualizes EA based on the DSM-IV criteria for substance abuse and dependence [10]. The EAI is a brief six-item tool that evaluates the six common symptoms of addictive behaviours: (i) salience; (ii) mood modification; (iii) tolerance; (iv) withdrawal symptoms; (v) social conflict; and (vi) relapse.

Over the years, different aetiopathogenetic hypotheses have emerged for EA. Several physiological hypotheses have been formulated, which involve beta-endorphins [28,29], the sympathetic nervous system [30], thermogenic regulation [31,32], and the catecholamine system [33].

Szabo proposed the cognitive appraisal hypothesis [34]. According to this theory, once habitual exercise is being used as a means of coping with stress, the individual comes to believe that exercise is a healthy way to deal with stress, and thus rationalizes the excessive amount of exercise. At the same time, other coping mechanisms are abandoned, resulting in the individual perceiving him- or herself as more vulnerable to stress, and this amplifies the negative psychological sensations associated with lack of exercise.

Finally, according to the hypothesis of affective regulation, exercise has a double effect on mood – it both increases positive affect and reduces negative affect [35]. However, these effects of physical exercise are only temporary, and are prone to the development of tolerance.

Freimuth's four-phase theory is the most widely recognized model for explaining the development of EA. In order of development, the four phases are recreational exercise, at-risk exercise, problematic exercise, and finally EA [36].

In addition, people with EA show abnormalities in their reward and inhibition systems, which may explain traits such as impulsiveness, loss of control, and impaired decision making. As has been demonstrated in the brains of people with substance addiction, hyperactivation of the reward system is manifested as enhanced activity in the prefrontal, limbic, and striatal areas, whereas a compromised inhibition system is manifested as lower amplitudes of N2 and P3 in the orbitofrontal-dorsolateral cortices [37]. These individuals need to exercise more in order to trigger the release of chemicals involved in the reward-seeking system.

Modern society ultimately acts as an important reinforcer of EA, as health and education organizations along with the media promote the beneficial effects of exercise and thinness. For this reason, EA is one of the most well-hidden behavioural addictions.

3.2 Comorbidities and Risk Factors

Sussman et al. have suggested that up to 25% of addicted people have more than one addictive disorder [38]. Research is sparse, but estimates indicate that 15–20% of individuals with exercise addiction are addicted to nicotine, alcohol, or illicit drugs [39], although not all of the studies demonstrated a relationship with alcohol or nicotine consumption [40]. Shopping addiction and internet addiction were identified as common among individuals with exercise addiction [19,41,42], whereas EA has been reported to be common among individuals with sex addiction [43].

As anticipated, there is a strong two-way link between EA and eating disorders [38]. Eating disorders are often accompanied by excessive levels of exercise; on the other hand, individuals affected by EA are often excessively concerned about their body image, weight, and strict dietary control [15,44–46]. Around 39–48% of people with eating disorders also suffer from EA [44,47].

Other risk factors for the development of EA are identifying strongly with people who are dedicated to exercise, having low self-esteem [48], or being anxious, impulsive, or extroverted [49]. Men and women are equally at risk, but in men the disorder is often primary, whereas in women it is often secondary [48,50].

In modern society, one factor with an important role in promoting the development of EA is the correlation between the ideal of a perfect body and success in life [51]. Excessive concerns about physical appearance can lead to the development of various appearance-related disorders, such as body dysmorphic disorder (BDD) [52,53] and muscle dysmorphia (MD) [54]. BDD is classified under 'Obsessive-Compulsive and Related Disorders' in DSM-5, and

MD is a specifier of it [55]. These disorders could either act as precursors or be secondary to other clinical conditions, such as eating disorders, mood disorders, and some addictive behaviours [56–59]. A study that used the EAI to measure the prevalence of EA in fitness settings across several European countries reported an EA prevalence of 11.7%. It also indicated a high risk of BDD (38.5%), mainly in women (47.2%). Equally high use of fitness-enhancing nutritional supplements (39.8%) was found. In women, an association between EA, appearance anxiety, and reduced self-esteem was identified [60].

BDD, formerly referred to as dysmorphophobia, is a serious psychiatric condition characterized by recurring and persistent concerns about an imaginary or minor defect in one's physical appearance; this may relate to a specific part of the body (e.g., nose, hair, freckles, breast size) or the body as a whole [53]. The concerns are intrusive, unwanted, and usually difficult to control [61,62], and include compulsive looking in the mirror, which affects most people with BDD [63]. BDD is underestimated and often undiagnosed [62]. When untreated, it affects most aspects of the affected person's life and ultimately global psychological well-being, as evidenced by its frequent association with severe depression, suicidal ideation, and functional impairment [64,65]. Individuals affected by EA and BDD are particularly at risk of using image- and performance-enhancing drugs (IPEDs), which are increasingly being sold on the Internet, where they are promoted by misleading marketing strategies. IPEDs include a wide range of products, which are described as having the potential to improve mental and physical functions. They include drugs for enhancing muscle structure and function, aiding weight loss, modifying the ageing process, promoting beauty and cosmetic appearance, and improving sexual performance and cognitive performance, among other functions. The IPED market is poorly regulated [66–68] and these products are frequently contaminated with biologically active ingredients, which means that they can pose significant health risks to those who use them [51,69–71].

Finally, social networks have contributed to the growing trend towards viewing physical exercise not as a path towards health, but as a means of achieving a desired appearance. This has been aided in particular by the continuous publication of photos and videos that show 'perfect' bodies, or the posting of messages that encourage training beyond human physical limits [72–75]. Such potentially harmful content could particularly affect more vulnerable individuals, such as teenagers and those with poor mental health who feel completely unable to attain such unrealistic ideals of beauty [76].

3.3 The COVID-19 Pandemic

On 31 December 2019, an outbreak of pneumonia of unknown aetiology was reported in the city of Wuhan, China. On 12 January 2020, Chinese researchers publicly shared the genetic sequence of the novel SARS-CoV-2 coronavirus

[77]. On 30 January 2020 the World Health Organization (WHO) declared that the outbreak of coronavirus disease (COVID-19) was a Public Health Emergency of International Relevance, and on 11 March 2020 the WHO announced that the COVID-19 outbreak had become a global pandemic [77].

SARS-CoV 2 is responsible for a severe acute respiratory syndrome [78] and is highly contagious; it can also affect the immune response and cause neurological complications [79,80].

From the start of the pandemic, governments and health authorities adopted various measures to limit the spread of the virus [81–83]. These included physical distancing (also known as social distancing), mandatory lockdown periods, and quarantine [84], all of which affected the lifestyles and daily habits of millions of people worldwide [85]. The measures resulted in numerous social [86,87] and economic [88–90] repercussions, as well as major consequences for the physical and mental health of the population [91].

Some of these measures have also been implemented during previous epidemics, such as severe acute respiratory syndrome (SARS), Middle East respiratory syndrome (MERS), and Ebola [92,93]. However, the global nature of the COVID-19 pandemic may have exacerbated the already known effects of both COVID-19 itself and the measures used to control it on the mental health of individuals [94], with many additional consequences [95].

The restrictions that were imposed facilitated a sedentary lifestyle and the development of unhealthy eating habits [96]. In addition to domestic confinement and reduced opportunities for engaging in outdoor activities, gyms, swimming pools, and fitness centres were often locked, and sporting events were postponed.

Video calls became the main means of communication both socially and for work, making satisfaction with one's appearance a factor of considerable importance [97]. In general, the amount of time spent online increased, including the time spent shopping [98].

3.4 New Risk Factors for the Development of Exercise Addiction

The radical changes that the COVID-19 pandemic caused in people's daily lives created fertile ground for the development of EA as well as other forms of addiction [99,100]. At the same time, individuals with EA, health-oriented people, and team exercisers were particularly affected by the limitation of their usual physical activity as a result of the measures that had been introduced to limit the spread of the virus [101]. These individuals might be compelled to significantly reduce their amount of daily exercise. However, people addicted to exercise were able to find alternative means of training, such as home exercises, or individual exercising that was allowed outdoors. Individuals who were exercising for health or therapeutic reasons were also keen to maintain their exercise regimes, in order to continue to manage their health disorder [102]. These individuals, consistent with the interactional model for EA [103], have a high risk of developing this disorder and therefore may not be able to reduce the amount of exercise that they engage in. Individuals who were addicted to team or group exercise may have experienced even greater difficulties, due to the closure of sports facilities and the inability to meet with other group members.

There is increasing evidence that regular exercise improves immunity in individuals of all ages, and that a physically active lifestyle can limit the ageing of the immune system, reducing the risk of contracting both transmissible diseases (e.g., viral and bacterial infections) and non-transmissible disorders (e.g., diabetes, hypertension, cancer) [104]. Therefore some individuals could push themselves to keep fit by exercising [105], and, particularly in an attempt to avoid transmission of COVID-19, some people might adapt this new lifestyle by exercising excessively and developing an unhealthy obsession with fitness. The lockdowns also offered more opportunities for over-exercising, due to home working with more flexible hours, having more free time, reduced opportunities to travel, and encouragement by public health organizations to exercise regularly.

At the same time, the lockdowns caused considerable stress, which can be attributed to a whole range of causes (e.g., domestic confinement, social and emotional isolation, crowded family homes, problems with childcare, and financial difficulties). In this context, physical activity could be a valid coping strategy, but with the possible risk of developing an addictive condition [106].

As stated earlier, individuals with AE often experience significant appearance anxiety, which could increase at a time when the widespread use of video calls made people's physical appearance one of the primary cues when interacting with others [97].

Similarly, spending more time online [98] could put people with EA at higher risk of purchasing and using IPEDs [76], which are advertised on the Internet as being capable of producing a dramatic improvement in physical appearance more quickly and safely than traditional methods [107–109].

Finally, the climate of great uncertainty regarding the physical, financial, social, and psychological impacts of the COVID-19 pandemic could also have contributed to the development or exacerbation of EA, as well as anxiety disorders and eating disorders [110]. This seems to be related to the intolerance of uncertainty that characterizes these disorders, and which is a transdiagnostic factor [111] that is believed to promote engagement in compulsive or safe behaviours [112,113] in response to perceived uncertainty. Intolerance of uncertainty might therefore contribute to the aetiology and maintenance of eating disorders [114,115] and might be associated with compulsive exercise [116], as both behaviours are perceived as useful for alleviating distress related to uncertainty [114].

3.5 The First Evidence of Exercise Addiction during the Pandemic

As yet the literature contains few studies about the role of the COVID-19 pandemic in inducing EA and influencing the aetiopathogenetic and pathological aspects of this condition. However, because of the enormous changes in people's lives that were caused by lockdowns and other restrictions, interest in this topic has recently been increasing [117].

An initial study was conducted in April 2020 in around 1,000 individuals aged 18–75 years (average age 33 years), all of whom had habitually exercised before the pandemic, from eight Spanish-speaking countries [101]. Changes in exercise volume were examined with regard to EA symptoms (severe, mild, or no EA symptoms), main reasons for exercise (health, skill, or social reasons), and forms of exercise (individual or group/team). The COVID-19-related decrease in exercise volume was approximately 50% in the sample. The risk of EA, assessed with the EAI, was 15.2%. Most (about 80%) of the participants exercised for health reasons. These users reported a smaller decrease in exercise volume than those who exercised for social reasons. The risk of EA was inversely related to changes in exercise volume, but this association disappeared after controlling for passion and perfectionism, which were measured with the revised Passion Scale (PS) [118] and the Frost Multidimensional Perfectionism Scale (FMPS) [119], respectively. The reported effect of COVID-19 on training did not differ between the EA symptom groups.

This pioneering study highlights the need to take into consideration the effects on physical and mental health that were caused by the restrictions imposed on physical activity. The smaller reduction in exercise volume among people who were exercising for health reasons could be explained in terms of the Health Belief Model [120]. According to this model, when a person feels threatened by morbidity, the greater the perceived threat, the more effort is made to overcome barriers and obstacles. Finally, the strong link between EA, passion [121,122], and perfectionism [21,123,124] is highlighted.

Another study, conducted on a sample of about 300 university students, examined the association between COVID-19 anxiety, intolerance of uncertainty, eating disorders, and compulsive exercise [110]. It was found that COVID-19-related anxiety and intolerance of uncertainty were associated with eating disorders, but not with compulsive exercise. In addition, intolerance of uncertainty moderated the associations between COVID-19-related anxiety, compulsive exercise, and eating disorders. COVID-19-related anxiety was more strongly related to compulsive exercise and eating disorders among individuals with lower intolerance of uncertainty.

Finally, between April and May 2020, a period of major restrictions across Europe, a survey was conducted on a large sample (3,161 individuals) of the general population recruited from seven different countries (the UK, Italy, Spain, Portugal, Lithuania, Hungary, and Japan) [76]. Participants were aged 15–80 years (average age 35 years). Only a few of them (1.6%) were professional athletes, and about 15% did not practise any type of exercise. The risk of EA was assessed with the EAI, appearance anxiety was measured with the Appearance Anxiety Inventory (AAI) [125], and self-compassion was assessed with the Self-Compassion Scale (SCS) [126]. The use of IPEDs was also investigated. Overall, 4.3% of the participants achieved a score indicative of EA with the EAI. The highest percentages were recorded in the UK and Spain, and among men. About 29% of the sample reported using IPEDs, mainly in Italy, the UK, and Lithuania, with 6.4% starting to use them during the lockdown. The use of IPEDs was also strongly associated with physical exercise – the consumption of IPEDs predicted the practice of physical exercise, and the risk of EA predicted the consumption of IPEDs. Significant levels of appearance anxiety were found among respondents from all countries, with 15.2% of the sample having levels that might indicate a risk of developing BDD. Italy, Japan, and Portugal were the countries with the highest number of people at risk for BDD. This risk was associated with less exercise among women and with higher levels of IPED consumption in the whole sample. Finally, there was a significant association between gender and self-compassion, with men presenting with higher levels of self-compassion. However, self-compassion did not show a significant relationship with engaging in physical exercise and the use of IPEDs.

This study found the highest percentage of EA among the general population. Considerable use of IPEDs was also identified, with higher rates of use than were reported in studies conducted before the pandemic. In addition, behaviours that are often thought to be aimed at maintaining or improving health, such as exercise or IPED consumption, could have become maladaptive during the period of restrictions imposed by the pandemic.

The relationship that emerges between physical exercise, anxiety about appearance, and the use of IPEDs needs to be highlighted, as easy online access to IPEDs and advertising strategies that recommend their consumption could lead to their use becoming a preferential strategy for shaping physical appearance.

Certain features of psychological functioning seemed to help to protect against EA and overuse of IPEDs. For example, self-compassion is an emotional self-regulation strategy that has been found to be associated with psychological benefits among young adults [127].

A study that focused on an Italian sample analysed which characteristics differentiated participants with EA (3.6%) from those without the condition [128]. Although the two groups did not differ in terms of demographic characteristics, type of sport practised, exercise routine, or whether or not they had had a pre-existing mental disorder, significant differences were observed in the perceived benefit of engaging in physical activity during the period of social distancing, in terms of the levels of appearance anxiety and self-compassion. The EA group reported perceiving a greater benefit due to training, and showed a higher level of appearance anxiety, a lower level of self-compassion, and significantly greater use of IPEDs.

Analysis of the factors that motivated the study subjects to exercise found that the EA group reported several factors significantly more often than did the non-risk group, namely physical wellness, psychological well-being, sexual attractiveness, and confidence in relationships. People with EA may view exercise as a source of physical and mental well-being and self-esteem, sometimes failing to consider the important effects of their way of exercising on their physical health, social relationships, and occupational functioning. Appearance anxiety emerged as a risk factor for EA, whereas self-compassion emerged as a protective factor. Finally, an association was found between EA and the use of IPEDs.

3.6 Conclusion

The restrictions that were imposed in an attempt to control the COVID-19 pandemic resulted in significant changes in the lives of the world's population. Many of these limitations act as risk factors for the development of EA. The initial studies of this subject support such a relationship. Longitudinal studies are therefore essential in order to deepen our knowledge of this subject. At the same time, mental health professionals need to recognise EA and implement practices to prevent the development of this disorder.

References

1   Waddington I. *Sport, Health and Drugs: A Critical Sociological Perspective.* Spoon Press, 2000.

2   Peluso MAM, Guerra de Andrade LHS. Physical activity and mental health: the association between exercise and mood. *Clinics* 2005; 60: 61–70.

3   Biddle SJH, Asare M. Physical activity and mental health in children and adolescents: a review of reviews. *Br J Sports Med* 2011; 45: 886–95.

4   Morgan WP. Negative addiction in runners. *Phys Sportsmed* 1979; 7: 56–70.

5   Griffiths M. Behavioural addiction: an issue for everybody? *Empl Couns Today* 1996; 8: 19–25.

6   Szabo A. *Addiction to Exercise: A Symptom or a Disorder?* Nova Science Publishers, 2010.

7   Thaxton L. Physiological and psychological effects of short-term addiction on habitual runners. *J Sport Psychol* 1982; 4: 73–80.

8   Hausenblas HA, Symons Downs D. How much is too much? The development and validation of the Exercise Addiction Scale. *Psychol Heal* 2002; 17: 387–404.

9   Symons Downs D, Hausenblas HA, Nigg CR. Factorial validity and psychometric examination of the Exercise Dependence Scale-Revised. *Meas Phys Educ Exerc Sci* 2004; 8: 183–201.

10 American Psychiatric Association. *Diagnostic and Statistical Manual of Mental Disorders*, 4th ed. American Psychiatric Association, 2000.

11 Albrecht U, Kirschner NE, Grüsser SM. Diagnostic instruments for behavioural addiction: an overview. *Psychosoc Med* 2007; 4: 1–11.

12 Di Forti M, Marconi A, Carra E et al. Proportion of patients in south London with first-episode psychosis attributable to use of high potency cannabis: a case-control study. *Lancet Psychiatry* 2015; 2: 233–8.

13 Grant JE, Potenza MN, Weinstein A, Gorelick DA. Introduction to behavioral addictions. *Am J Drug Alcohol Abuse* 2010; 36: 233–41.

14 Bamber D, Carroll D, Cockerill IM, Rodgers S. "It's exercise or nothing": a qualitative analysis of exercise dependence. *Br J Sports Med* 2000; 34: 423–30.

15 Blaydon MJ, Lindner KJ. Eating disorders and exercise dependence in triathletes. *Eat Disord* 2002; 10: 49–60.

16 De Coverley Veale DMW. Exercise dependence. *Br J Addict* 1987; 82: 735–40.

17 Berczik K, Szabó A, Griffiths MD et al. Exercise addiction: symptoms, diagnosis, epidemiology, and etiology. *Subst Use Misuse* 2012; 47: 403–17.

18 Slay HA, Hayaki J, Napolitano MA, Brownell KD. Motivations for running and eating attitudes in obligatory versus nonobligatory runners. *Int J Eat Disord* 1998; 23: 267–75.

19 Lejoyeux M, Avril M, Richoux C, Embouazza H, Nivoli F. Prevalence of exercise dependence and other behavioral addictions among clients of a Parisian fitness room. *Compr Psychiatry* 2008; 49: 353–8.

20 Allegre B, Therme P, Griffiths M. Individual factors and the context of physical activity in exercise dependence: a prospective study of "ultra-marathoners." *Int J Ment Health Addict* 2007; 5: 233–43.

21 Schipfer M, Stoll O. OR-77: Exercise-Addiction/Exercise-Commitment-Model (EACOM). *J Behav Addict* 2015; 4: 35–7.

22 Terry A, Szabo A, Griffiths M. The Exercise Addiction Inventory: a new brief screening tool. *Addict Res Theory* 2004; 12: 489–99.

23 Hausenblas HA, Fallon EA. Relationship among body image, exercise behavior, and exercise dependence symptoms. *Int J Eat Disord* 2002; 32: 179–85.

24 Griffiths M. A "components" model of addiction within a biopsychosocial framework. *J Subst Use* 2005; 10: 191–7.

25 Szabo A, Griffiths MD. Exercise addiction in British sport science students. *Int J Ment Health Addict* 2007; 5: 25–8.

26 Mónok K, Berczik K, Urbán R et al. Psychometric properties and concurrent validity of two exercise addiction measures: a population wide study. *Psychol Sport Exerc* 2012; 13: 739–46.

27 Griffiths MD, Urbán R, Demetrovics Z et al. A cross-cultural re-evaluation of the Exercise Addiction Inventory (EAI) in five countries. *Sport Med Open* 2015; 1: 1–7.

28 Goldberg A. *The Sports Mind: A Workbook of Mental Skills for Athletes.* Competitive Advantage, 1988.

29 Farrell PA, Gates WK, Maksud MG, Morgan WP. Increases in plasma β-endorphin/β-lipotropin immunoreactivity after treadmill running in humans. *J Appl Physiol Respir Environ Exerc Physiol* 1982; 52: 1245–9.

30 Thompson JK, Blanton P. Energy conservation and exercise dependence: a sympathetic arousal hypothesis. *Med Sci Sports Exerc* 1987; 19: 91–9.

31 DeVries HA. Tranquilizer effect of exercise: a critical review. *Phys Sportsmed* 1981; 9: 47–55.

32 Morgan WP, O'Connor PJ. Exercise and mental health. In: Dishman RK, ed. *Exercise Adherence: Its Impact on Public Health.* Human Kinetics, 1988: 91–121.

33 Cousineau D, Ferguson RJ, de Champlain J et al. Catecholamines in coronary sinus during exercise in man before and after training. *J Appl Physiol Respir Environ Exerc Physiol* 1977; 43: 801–6.

34 Szabo A. The impact of exercise deprivation on well-being of habitual exercises. *Aust J Sci Med Sport* 1995; 27: 68–75.

35 Hamer M, Karageorghis CI. Psychobiological mechanisms of exercise dependence. *Sports Med* 2007; 37: 477–84.

36 Freimuth M, Moniz S, Kim SR. Clarifying exercise addiction: differential diagnosis, co-occurring disorders, and phases of addiction. *Int J Environ Res Public Health* 2011; 8: 4069–81.

37 Huang QIN, Huang J, Chen Y et al. Overactivation of the reward system and deficient inhibition in exercise addiction. *Med Sci Sports Exerc* 2019; 51: 1918–27.

38 Sussman S, Lisha N, Griffiths M. Prevalence of the addictions: a problem of the majority or the minority? *Eval Heal Prof* 2011; 34: 3–56.

39 Aidman EV, Woollard S. The influence of self-reported exercise addiction on acute emotional and physiological responses to brief exercise deprivation. *Psychol Sport Exerc* 2003; 4: 225–36.

40 Allegre B, Souville M, Therme P, Griffiths M. Definitions and measures of exercise dependence. *Addict Res Theory* 2006; 14: 631–46.

41 Di Nicola M, Tedeschi D, De Risio L et al. Co-occurrence of alcohol use disorder and behavioral addictions: relevance of impulsivity and craving. *Drug Alcohol Depend* 2015; 148: 118–25.

42   Müller A, Loeber S, Söchtig J, Te Wildt B, De Zwaan M. Risk for exercise dependence, eating disorder pathology, alcohol use disorder and addictive behaviors among clients of fitness centers. *J Behav Addict* 2015; 4: 273–80.

43   Carnes PJ, Murray RE, Charpentier L. Bargains with chaos: sex addicts and addiction interaction disorder. *Sex Addict Compulsivity* 2005; 12: 79–120.

44   Klein DA, Bennett AS, Schebendach J et al. Exercise "addiction" in anorexia nervosa: model development and pilot data. *CNS Spectr* 2004; 9: 531–7.

45   Lyons HA, Cromey R. Compulsive jogging: exercise dependence and associated disorder of eating. *Ulster Med J* 1989; 58: 100–2.

46   Sundgot-Borgen J. Eating disorders in female athletes. *Sports Med* 1994; 17: 176–88.

47   Bamber DJ, Cockerill IM, Rodgers S, Carroll D. Diagnostic criteria for exercise dependence in women. *Br J Sports Med* 2003; 37: 393–400.

48   Bruno A, Quattrone D, Scimeca G et al. Unraveling exercise addiction: the role of narcissism and self-esteem. *J Addict* 2014; 2014: 1–6.

49   Hausenblas HA, Giacobbi PR. Relationship between exercise dependence symptoms and personality. *Pers Individ Dif* 2004; 36: 1265–73.

50   Cunningham HE, Pearman S, Brewerton TD. Conceptualizing primary and secondary pathological exercise using available measures of excessive exercise. *Int J Eat Disord* 2016; 49: 778–92.

51   Mooney R, Simonato P, Ruparelia R et al. The use of supplements and performance and image enhancing drugs in fitness settings: an exploratory cross-sectional investigation in the United Kingdom. *Hum Psychopharmacol* 2017; 32: e2619.

52   Al-Sarraf A, Khatib Y, Corazza O. The interaction between skin and mind: the case of body dysmorphic disorder. *Res Adv Psychiatry* 2018; 5: 38–42.

53   Buhlmann U, Glaesmer H, Mewes R et al. Updates on the prevalence of body dysmorphic disorder: a population-based survey. *Psychiatry Res* 2010; 178: 171–5.

54   Sandgren SS, Lavallee D. Muscle dysmorphia research neglects DSM-5 diagnostic criteria. *J Loss Trauma* 2018; 23: 211–43.

55   American Psychiatric Association. *Diagnostic and Statistical Manual of Mental Disorders*, 5th ed. American Psychiatric Association, 2013.

56   Altamura C, Paluello MM, Mundo E, Medda S, Mannu P. Clinical and subclinical body dysmorphic disorder. *Eur Arch Psychiatry Clin Neurosci* 2001; 251: 105–8.

57   Beucke JC, Sepulcre J, Buhlmann U et al. Degree connectivity in body dysmorphic disorder and relationships with obsessive and compulsive symptoms. *Eur Neuropsychopharmacol* 2016; 26: 1657–66.

58   Leone JE, Sedory EJ, Gray KA. Recognition and treatment of muscle dysmorphia and related body image disorders. *J Athl Train* 2005; 40: 352–9.

59   Murray SB, Rieger E, Hildebrandt T et al. A comparison of eating, exercise, shape, and weight related symptomatology in males with muscle dysmorphia and anorexia nervosa. *Body Image* 2012; 9: 193–200.

60   Corazza O, Simonato P, Demetrovics Z et al. The emergence of exercise addiction, body dysmorphic disorder, and other image-related psychopathological correlates in fitness settings: a cross sectional study. *PLoS ONE* 2019; 14: e0213060.

61   Silver J, Farrants J. 'I once stared at myself in the mirror for eleven hours.' Exploring mirror gazing in participants with body dysmorphic disorder. *J Health Psychol* 2016; 21: 2647–57.

62   Bewley A. The neglected psychological aspects of skin disease. *BMJ* 2017; 6: j3208.

63   Veale D, Riley S. Mirror, mirror on the wall, who is the ugliest of them all? The psychopathology of mirror gazing in body dysmorphic disorder. *Behav Res Ther* 2001; 39: 1381–93.

64   Soler PT, Ferreira CMH, Novaes J da S, Fernandes HM. Body dysmorphic disorder: characteristics, psychopathology, clinical associations, and influencing factors. In: Gaze DC, ed. *Pathophysiology: Altered Physiological States*. IntechOpen, 2018: 3–22.

65   Veale D, Bewley A. Body dysmorphic disorder. *BMJ* 2015; 350: h2278.

66   Corazza O, Roman-Urrestarazu A. *Novel Psychoactive Substances: Policy, Economics and Drug. Regulation.* Springer, 2017.

67   Reuter P, Pardo B. Can new psychoactive substances be regulated effectively? An assessment of the British Psychoactive Substances Bill. *Addiction* 2017; 112: 25–31.

68   Heinrich J. *Dietary Supplements For Weight Loss: Limited Federal Oversight Has Focused More on Marketing than on Safety.* GAO-02-985T, 2002. www.gao.gov/products/GAO-02-985T

69   Graham MR, Ryan P, Baker JS et al. Counterfeiting in performance- and image-enhancing drugs. *Drug Test Anal* 2009; 1: 135–42.

70   Thevis M, Schrader Y, Thomas A et al. Analysis of confiscated black market drugs using chromatographic and mass spectrometric approaches. *J Anal Toxicol* 2008; 32: 232–40.

71   Van de Ven K, Maher L, Wand H et al. Health risk and health seeking behaviours among people who inject performance and image enhancing drugs who access needle syringe programs in Australia. *Drug Alcohol Rev* 2018; 37: 837–46.

72   Barry CT, Doucette H, Loflin DC, Rivera-Hudson N, Herrington LL. "Let me take a selfie": associations between self-photography, narcissism, and self-esteem. *Psychol Pop Media Cult* 2017; 6: 48–60.

73   Mabe AG, Forney KJ, Keel PK. Do you "like" my photo? Facebook use maintains eating disorder risk. *Int J Eat Disord* 2014; 47: 516–23.

74   Meier EP, Gray J. Facebook photo activity associated with body image disturbance in adolescent girls. *Cyberpsychol Behav Soc Netw* 2014; 17: 199–206.

75 Simpson CC, Mazzeo SE. Skinny is not enough: a content analysis of fitspiration on Pinterest. *Health Commun* 2017; 32: 560–7.

76 Dores AR, Carvalho IP, Burkauskas J et al. Exercise and use of enhancement drugs at the time of the COVID-19 pandemic: a multicultural study on coping strategies during self-isolation and related risks. *Front Psychiatry* 2021; 12: 648501.

77 World Health Organization (WHO). *Archived: WHO Timeline - COVID-19*. World Health Organization, 2020. www.who.int/news/item/27-04-2020-who-timeline—covid-19

78 Xu Z, Li S, Tian S, Li H, Kong LQ. Full spectrum of COVID-19 severity still being depicted. *Lancet* 2020; 395: 947–8.

79 Cothran TP, Kellman S, Singh S et al. A brewing storm: the neuropsychological sequelae of hyperinflammation due to COVID-19. *Brain Behav Immun* 2020; 88: 957-8.

80 Ellul MA, Benjamin L, Singh B et al. Neurological associations of COVID-19. *Lancet Neurol* 2020; 19: 767–83.

81 Ferguson NM, Laydon D, Nedjati-Gilani G et al. *Impact of Non-Pharmaceutical Interventions (NPIs) to Reduce COVID-19 Mortality and Healthcare Demand.* Imperial College London, 2020. www.imperial.ac.uk/mrc-global-infectious-disease-analysis/covid-19/report-9-impact-of-npis-on-covid-19/

82 Mendes-Santos C, Andersson G, Weiderpass E, Santana R. Mitigating COVID-19 impact on the Portuguese population mental health: the opportunity that lies in digital mental health. *Front Public Heal* 2020; 8: 553345.

83 Wise T, Zbozinek TD, Michelini G, Hagan CC, Mobbs D. Changes in risk perception and self-reported protective behaviour during the first week of the COVID-19 pandemic in the United States. *R Soc Open Sci* 2020; 7: 200742.

84 Santana R, Rocha J, Soares P, Sousa J. *Os Momentos das Políticas de Saúde no Combate ao COVID-19.* Escola Nacional de Saúde Publica (ENSP), 2020. https://barometro-covid-19.ensp.unl.pt/wp-content/uploads/2020/04/osmomentosdaspoliticasdesaudenocombateaocovid19–26.03.2020.pdf

85 Ammar A, Trabelsi K, Brach M et al. Effects of home confinement on mental health and lifestyle behaviours during the COVID-19 outbreak: insights from the ECLB-COVID19 multicentre study. *Biol Sport* 2021; 38: 9–21.

86 Dores AR, Geraldo A, Carvalho IP, Barbosa F. The use of new digital information and communication technologies in psychological counseling during the COVID-19 pandemic. *Int J Environ Res Public Health* 2020; 17: 7663.

87 Prime H, Wade M, Browne DT. Risk and resilience in family well-being during the COVID-19 pandemic. *Am Psychol* 2020; 75: 631–43.

88 Bluedorn J, Gopinath GSD. An early view of the economic impact of the pandemic in 5 charts. IMFBlog, International Monetary Fund, 2020. https://blogs.imf.org/2020/04/06/an-early-view-of-the-economic-impact-of-the-pandemic-in-5-charts/

89 Maital S, Barzani E. *The Global Economic Impact of COVID-19: A Summary of Research.* Samuel Neaman Institute, 2020. www.neaman.org.il/EN/The-Global-Economic-Impact-of-COVID-19-A-Summary-of-Research

90 Stiglitz JE, Shiller RJ, Gopinath G et al. *How the Economy Will Look After the Coronavirus Pandemic.* Foreign Policy, 2020. https://foreignpolicy.com/2020/04/15/how-the-economy-will-look-after-the-coronavirus-pandemic

91 Alzueta E, Perrin P, Baker FC et al. How the COVID-19 pandemic has changed our lives: a study of psychological correlates across 59 countries. *J Clin Psychol* 2021; 77: 556–70.

92 Jeong H, Yim HW, Song YJ et al. Mental health status of people isolated due to Middle East Respiratory Syndrome. *Epidemiol Health* 2016; 38: e2016048.

93 Brooks SK, Webster RK, Smith LE et al. The psychological impact of quarantine and how to reduce it: rapid review of the evidence. *Lancet* 2020; 345: 912–20.

94 Horesh D, Brown AD. Traumatic stress in the age of COVID-19: a call to close critical gaps and adapt to new realities. *Psychol Trauma* 2020; 12: 331–5.

95 Holmes EA, O'Connor RC, Perry VH et al. Multidisciplinary research priorities for the COVID-19 pandemic: a call for action for mental health science. *Lancet Psychiatry* 2020; 7: 547–60.

96 Ammar A, Brach M, Trabelsi K et al. Effects of COVID-19 home confinement on eating behaviour and physical activity: results of the ECLB-COVID19 international online survey. *Nutrients* 2020; 12: 1583.

97 Pfund GN, Hill PL, Harriger J. Video chatting and appearance satisfaction during COVID-19: appearance comparisons and self-objectification as moderators. *Int J Eat Disord* 2020; 53: 2038–43.

98 Zamboni L, Carli S, Marika B et al. COVID-19 lockdown: impact on online gambling, online shopping, web navigation and online pornography. *J Public Health Res* 2021; 10: 97–102.

99 Czeisler MÉ, Ma RIL, Petrosky E et al. Mental health, substance use, and suicidal ideation during the COVID-19 pandemic — United States, June 24–30, 2020. *Morb Mortal Wkly Rep* 2020; 69: 1049–57.

100 Martinotti G, Alessi MC, Di Natale C et al. Psychopathological burden and quality of life in substance users during the COVID-19 lockdown period in Italy. *Front Psychiatry* 2020; 11:1–8.

101 De la Vega R, Almendros LJ, Barquín RR et al. Exercise addiction during the COVID-19 pandemic: an international study confirming the need for considering passion and perfectionism. *Int J Ment Health Addict* 2022; 20: 1159–70.

102 Szabo A, Kovacsik R. When passion appears, exercise addiction disappears: should hundreds of studies not considering passion be revisited? *Swiss J Psychol* 2019; 78: 137–42.

103 Egorov AY, Szabo A. The exercise paradox: an interactional model for a clearer conceptualization of exercise addiction. *J Behav Addict* 2013; 2: 199–208.

104 Campbell JP, Turner JE. Debunking the myth of exercise-induced immune suppression: redefining the impact of exercise on immunological health across the lifespan. *Front Immunology* 2018; 9: 648.

105 Chamorro-Viña C, Fernandez-Del-Valle M, Tacón AM. Excessive exercise and immunity: the J-shaped curve. In: McComb JJ, Norman R, Zumwalt M, eds. *The Active Female: Health Issues Throughout the Lifespan*, 2nd ed. Springer, 2014: 357–72.

106 Lim MA. Exercise addiction and COVID-19-associated restrictions. *J Ment Health* 2021; 30: 135-7.

107 Molinero O, Marquez S. Use of nutritional supplements in sports: risks, knowledge, and behavioural-related factors. *Nutr Hosp* 2009; 24: 128–34.

108 Müller RK. History of doping and doping control. In: Thieme D, Hemmersbach P, eds. *Doping in Sports: Biochemical Principles, Effects and Analysis*. Springer, 2010: 1–23.

109 Kamber M, Mullis PE. The worldwide fight against doping: from the beginning to the world anti-doping agency. *Endocrinol Metab Clin North Am* 2010; 39: 1–9.

110 Scharmer C, Martinez K, Gorrell S et al. Eating disorder pathology and compulsive exercise during the COVID-19 public health emergency: examining risk associated with COVID-19 anxiety and intolerance of uncertainty. *Int J Eat Disord* 2020; 53: 2049–54.

111 Mahoney AEJ, McEvoy PM. Trait versus situation-specific intolerance of uncertainty in a clinical sample with anxiety and depressive disorders. *Cogn Behav Ther* 2012; 41: 26–39.

112 Boswell JF, Thompson-Hollands J, Farchione TJ, Barlow DH. Intolerance of uncertainty: a common factor in the treatment of emotional disorders. *J Clin Psychol* 2013; 69: 630–45.

113 Holaway RM, Heimberg RG, Coles ME. A comparison of intolerance of uncertainty in analogue obsessive-compulsive disorder and generalized anxiety disorder. *J Anxiety Disord* 2006; 20: 158–74.

114 Brown M, Robinson L, Campione GC et al. Intolerance of uncertainty in eating disorders: a systematic review and meta-analysis. *Eur Eat Disord Rev* 2017; 25: 329–43.

115 Kesby A, Maguire S, Brownlow R, Grisham JR. Intolerance of uncertainty in eating disorders: an update on the field. *Clin Psychol Rev* 2017; 56: 94–105.

116 Scharmer C, Reilly EE, Gorrell S, Anderson DA. Establishing a link between compulsive exercise and intolerance of uncertainty to inform intervention development. Paper presented at the University of California San Diego 4th Annual Eating Disorders Conference, 27–28 February 2020, San Diego.

117 Juwono ID, Szabo A. 100 cases of exercise addiction: more evidence for a widely researched but rarely identified dysfunction. *Int J Ment Health Addict* 2021; 19: 1799–811.

118 Marsh HW, Vallerand RJ, Lafreniére MAK et al. Passion: does one scale fit all? Construct validity of two-factor passion scale and psychometric invariance over different activities and languages. *Psychol Assess* 2013; 25: 796–809.

119 Frost RO, Marten PA. Perfectionism and evaluative threat. *Cogn Ther Res* 1990; 14: 559–72.

120 Rosenstock IM. Historical origins of the health belief model. *Health Educ Behav* 1974; 2: 328–35.

121 Kovacsik R, Griffiths MD, Pontes HM et al. The role of passion in exercise addiction, exercise volume, and exercise intensity in long-term exercisers. *Int J Ment Health Addict* 2019; 17: 1389–400.

122 Kovacsik R, Soós I, De la Vega R, Ruíz-Barquín R, Szabo A. Passion and exercise addiction: healthier profiles in team than in individual sports. *Int J Sport Exerc Psychol* 2020; 18: 176–86.

123 Birche J, Griffiths MD, Kasos K, Demetrovics Z, Szabo A. Exercise addiction and personality: a two-decade systematic review of the empirical literature (1995–2016). *Balt J Sport Heal Sci* 2017; 3: 19–33.

124 Curran T, Hill AP, Jowett GE, Mallinson SH. The relationship between multidimensional perfectionism and passion in junior athletes. *Int J Sport Psychol* 2014; 45: 369–84.

125 Veale D, Eshkevari E, Kanakam N et al. The Appearance Anxiety Inventory: validation of a process measure in the treatment of body dysmorphic disorder. *Behav Cogn Psychother* 2014; 42: 605–16.

126 Neff KD. The development and validation of a scale to measure self-compassion. *Neuropsychopharmacology* 2003; 2: 223–50.

127 Castilho P, Gouveia JP. Auto-Compaixão: estudo da validação da versão portuguesa da Escala da Auto-Compaixão e da sua relação com as experiências adversas na infância, a comparação social e a psicopatologia [Self-Compassion: study of the validation of the Portuguese version of the Self-Compassion Scale and its relationship with adverse childhood experiences, social comparison and psychopathology]. *Psychologica* 2011; 54: 203–30.

128 Ceci F, Di Carlo F, Burkauskas J et al. Physical activity and exercise addiction during the Covid-19 pandemic in Italy. *Int J Ment Health Addict* 2022. DOI: https:// doi.org/10.1007/s11469-022-00815-z

Chapter

Excessive Exercise and Image- and Performance-Enhancing Drug Use Among Sports Disciplines, and the Role of Mind–Body Training

Hironobu Fujiwara and Mami Shibata

4.1 The Evolution of Sport in Society, and Related Health Benefits and Risks

Exercise is widely known to have positive effects on both body and mind. In recent years, the number and variety of different sports disciplines have been expanding. For example, new styles of gyms, such as those specialized for CrossFit (a high-density workout programme that consists of three types of exercise – weightlifting, callisthenics, and aerobic exercise) are being established. For disabled individuals and older adults, the concept of 'esports' has recently been shown to have health benefits, in addition to its initial purpose as a leisure pursuit.

Esports is a potentially suitable method of rehabilitation in the fields of welfare and medical care because it can be played by individuals of any age or ability. For example, in Japan the spread of esports to the elderly is aimed at promoting health (e.g., by maintaining and improving cognitive function) [1], and in Korea a patient with muscular dystrophy became a top professional gamer [2,3].

Although the health-promoting effects of exercise are widely known, it has been pointed out that excessive exercise can also potentially damage health, when it is associated with problems such as overtraining syndrome and burnout. Health impairment caused by excessive exercise could be viewed as a kind of 'behavioural addiction' from a psychiatric, psychological, and physical health perspective [4,5]. Behavioural addiction is a non-drug-related form of addiction, examples of which include addiction related to gambling, internet use, gaming, food intake, sex, and shopping, and it has potentially harmful effects on health [6–9].

In relation to behavioural addiction, concern has been expressed about excessive exercise and its association with the abuse of image- and performance-enhancing drugs (IPEDs) among people who habitually engage in sports activities. Excessive exercise is thought to be linked to psychological states, including anxiety about appearance, body weight, or muscle mass, as well as interest in physical and mental health. Investigations of how the relationship between excessive exercise and psychological state varies among a whole range of different sports disciplines may enable the development of tailor-made ways to address the risk of excessive exercise within each sports discipline. Furthermore, it is important to determine the relationship between excessive exercise and IPED use when assessing the risk of 'cross addiction' – that is, a state in which there are two comorbid addictions, and each addiction perpetuates the other. The consumption of IPEDs, which are used daily by athletes, can potentially result in a form of over-enhancement, such as that seen in doping. It has been reported that the use of IPEDs is related to a tendency to exercise excessively [4]. Therefore it is important to investigate how the relationship between excessive exercise and IPED use varies among different sports disciplines.

4.2 Excessive Exercise and the Use of IPEDs Across Different Sports

Since 2020, many aspects of our lifestyle, including our exercise habits, have been changing dramatically due to the coronavirus disease (COVID-19) pandemic. However, it has not yet been clarified whether the various sports disciplines differ with regard to the prevalence of excessive exercising and also its association with IPED use during the COVID-19 pandemic. The authors of this chapter were involved in conducting an online survey to investigate this [10]. They hypothesized that the pattern of engaging in exercise and using IPEDs as a coping strategy might have changed significantly across various sports disciplines during the pandemic. Endurance athletes (e.g., ball game players), fitness centre attendees, and those engaged in power disciplines had already been shown to be at higher risk of excessive exercising prior to the pandemic [11]. A relationship was also found between excessive exercise and different types of psychological functioning, such as appearance anxiety [4,12] and self-compassion [13]. Differences in the use of IPEDs also emerged across different sports. Higher scores on the Appearance Anxiety Inventory (AAI) might have indicated that individuals were more concerned about and critical of their physical appearance during the lockdown. Higher scores on the Self-Compassion Scale (SCS) – a measure of a concept that includes kindness to oneself, common humanity, and mindfulness [13], which is needed as a coping strategy when individuals are facing difficulties – might play a role in developing a safer and more positive attitude towards a challenging situation, and in mitigating excessive exercise and IPED use.

A total of 2,295 individuals participated in the online survey. They were engaged in a variety of sports, mainly generic workouts, walking, weightlifting, running, yoga, fighting sports (e.g., boxing, kickboxing, martial arts), swimming, dance, martial arts, cycling, ball sports, Budo, and CrossFit. For the purposes of this study, the term 'generic workout' included individuals who engaged in some general running, weightlifting, and other free body exercises to keep fit and tone their muscles. The term 'martial arts' included oriental (non-Western cultural style) fighting sports such as Kendo, Judo, Aikido, Karate, Taekwondo, Brazilian jiu-jitsu, Muay Thai, Wushu, Tai Chi, and Capoeira, and the term 'Budo' included martial arts of Japanese origin, such as Kendo, Aikido, Judo, and Karate.

The results of the study can be summarized briefly as follows. As shown in Table 4.1, the Exercise Addiction Inventory (EAI) score for walking was considerably lower than the EAI scores for the other sports disciplines, whereas weightlifting and CrossFit had higher EAI scores than the other sports disciplines. Thus the tendency to exercise excessively is lower in walking, whereas it is higher in weightlifting and CrossFit. With regard to appearance anxiety, Budo and cycling had the lowest AAI scores, whereas weightlifting, CrossFit, and dance had the highest AAI scores. Although there was no significant difference in SCS scores among the sport disciplines, cycling had the highest SCS score.

There was significant variation in the percentage of IPED users among the different sports disciplines. Specifically, IPED use was significantly higher in weightlifting (61.1%) and CrossFit (60.3%) than in other disciplines, whereas it was significantly lower in walking (24.5%) than in other disciplines. In addition, high EAI and AAI scores were found to be significantly correlated with IPED use among individuals who exercised regularly. As shown in Figure 4.1, sports disciplines were categorized into three groups according to the EAI score: (i) high EAI group, (ii) low EAI group; and (iii) others. Weightlifting and CrossFit corresponded to the high EAI group. Only walking corresponded to the low EAI group. These results confirm previous findings which suggested that endurance athletes, ball game players, fitness centre attendees, and those engaged in power disciplines have a high risk of exercising excessively [11]. It is worth noting that among the sports disciplines with a high EAI score, weightlifting and CrossFit also showed higher IPED use. Conversely, walking, which was in the low EAI group, was significantly associated with a lower rate of IPED use. Individuals who practise weightlifting often aim to increase strength and muscle hypertrophy. However, if the training becomes obsessive and compulsive, it can lead to muscle dysmorphia [14,15]. Since CrossFit is recognized as a type of high-intensity functional training associated with a high risk of excessive exercising [16,17], this sport could have some traits in common with weightlifting [18]. Consequently, it could be suggested that the observation that 'the higher the EAI score, the higher the IPED use' indicates that excessive exercise is associated with the risk of cross addiction with substance intake.

Table 4.1 Scores on the Exercise Addiction Inventory (EAI), Appearance Anxiety Inventory (AAI), and Self-Compassion Scale (SCS) for each sports discipline

Sports discipline	EAI score	
Running	17.79±3.46	F = 8.11,
Swimming	16.98±3.28	p < 0.001
Fighting sports	17.70±3.72	
Martial arts	17.76±3.38	
Budo	17.36±3.04	
Cycling	16.44±3.58	
Ball sports	17.62±4.49	
Generic workout	17.11±3.75	
Weightlifting	18.02±3.70	
CrossFit	19.06±3.86	
Mountain climbing	17.89±3.14	
Yoga	16.65±3.86	
Walking	15.77±3.83	
Tennis	17.74±3.26	
Other	16.54±4.07	
Dance	17.41±3.64	

Sports discipline	AAI score	
None	16.65±5.59	F = 6.98
Running	16.40±5.57	p < 0.001
Swimming	15.69±4.81	
Fighting sports	15.51±5.07	
Martial arts	15.75±5.23	
Budo	14.60±4.37	
Cycling	14.29±4.41	
Ball sports	16.49±4.95	
Generic workout	17.19±5.42	
Weightlifting	18.35±5.93	
CrossFit	18.46±5.53	
Mountain climbing	15.08±5.41	
Yoga	16.18±4.76	
Walking	16.36±5.64	
Tennis	14.97±4.63	
Other	16.85±6.60	
Dance	18.09±6.16	

Sports discipline	SCS score	
None	30.54±5.78	F = 1.64
Running	31.18±6.04	p = 0.052
Swimming	31.42±5.94	
Fighting sports	31.40±5.53	
Martial arts	31.20±5.64	
Budo	31.33±5.57	
Cycling	32.82±5.83	
Ball sports	30.00±6.25	

Table 4.1 (cont.)

Sports discipline	SCS score
Generic workout	30.87±5.96
Weightlifting	30.27±6.10
CrossFit	31.49±5.54
Mountain climbing	31.46±5.67
Yoga	31.70±5.70
Walking	31.11±6.10
Tennis	31.34±6.22
Other	30.58±6.59
Dance	30.46±7.08

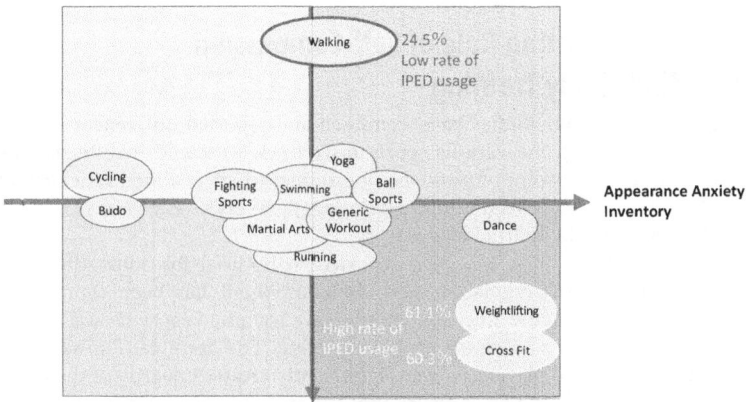

Exercise Addiction Inventory

Figure 4.1 Schematic representation of the features of the Exercise Addiction Inventory (EAI) and Appearance Anxiety Inventory (AAI) for each sports discipline.

In addition, because of the ready availability of IPEDs online (12.2% of those who used IPEDs had purchased them online), it may be necessary to assume a risk of cross addiction with excessive internet use, as well as excessive exercise and IPED abuse. Although there was no significant difference in self-compassion among sports disciplines in this investigation, the authors suggested that self-compassion needs further investigation. Self-compassion was defined as a psychological construct that involves treating oneself with the kindness and compassion that is given to others when faced with pain or difficulty, focusing on Buddhist principles that are rooted in Eastern philosophy [19]. The SCS has three conceptual components, namely self-kindness, a sense of common humanity, and mindfulness [13].

Only a few studies have examined the relationship between self-compassion and sports. High levels of self-compassion are associated with strong coping skills and high motivation of athletes to engage in sports [20]. Furthermore, high levels of self-compassion are inversely related to the risk of substance use disorders, such as addiction to alcohol or cannabis [21,22]. The finding of high SCS scores in swimmers led Barczak and Eklund to suggest that self-compassion influenced swimmers' performance, leading to a positive coping and motivational mindset [20]. One possible explanation is that swimming itself acts as a strategy for coping with stress in daily life, which is influenced by self-compassion. As these studies have reported, it is conceivable that self-compassion could contribute to maintaining or promoting mental health, such as coping skills or impulse control, enabling those engaged in the different sports disciplines to resist substance abuse.

4.3 The Mediating Role of Self-Compassion and Mind–Body Training

Although to date no studies have examined and reported differences in self-compassion among the various sports disciplines, we could investigate this issue from the viewpoint of mind–body training, which is aimed at achieving greater integration between mind (psychology) and body (exercise) [23]. This is often practised by martial arts players.

Mind–body training has been reported to be used for cultivating self-compassion and self-regulation [24]. In addition, it has been found that individuals who practise intensive mind–body training report several cognitive health benefits as a result of their training. For example, Fujiwara has reported that Kendo players showed significantly greater integrity of the brain functional network, which involves motivational function in attention processing [25].

In the sports disciplines within the main study described earlier, Budo and yoga had relatively high SCS scores compared with other sports disciplines, and were thought to share several characteristics. The mind–body integrated approach is one of the common features of combining mentality with physical training – that is, mind–body training emphasizes the importance of breathing control [26]. In this sense, both Budo and yoga differ from other sports training. Yoga, which is an ancient Indian mind–body integrated strategy for health promotion, utilizes specific postures (*asana*) and regulation of breathing (*pranayama*). It is useful for enhancing the mind's capacity to affect bodily function and symptoms [27] as an alternative therapy. One study has shown that yoga reduces anxiety and depression [28–30]. In Budo, aspects of both physical exercise and the individual's mindset are emphasized, particularly the concept of 'mind–body unity' [25,31], and the discipline is based on the concepts of Zen Buddhism [23]. A neuroimaging study found evidence that Budo was associated with better functioning in the processing of motivation as mind–body training [25]. In addition, the regulation of breathing (*Chosoku*), together with arranging the mind (*Choshin*), play an important role in Budo and meditation. This includes *Zazen*, which is practised in Zen Buddism [32]. In relation to the finding of high SCS scores in swimmers, Barczak and Eklund suggested that self-compassion influenced swimmers' performance, resulting in the development of positive coping and motivational mindsets [20], although there was no direct evidence for a commonality among Budo, yoga, and swimming. One possible explanation is that swimming itself might act as a coping strategy for stress in daily life, which is influenced by self-compassion. Thus the fostering of self-compassion might be important when establishing exercise habits for the benefit of mental health, particularly in the context of prevention of excessive performance enhancement by supplement use.

4.4 Conclusion

In general, the research described in this chapter has shown that excessive exercise could potentially be associated with excessive IPED use, which may have exacerbated negative outcomes during the COVID-19 pandemic. It is important to pay attention to the risks associated with IPED consumption, particularly among individuals with traits of excessive exercising or appearance anxiety who engage in sports disciplines that demand high-intensity functional training, as it was in those disciplines that individuals were found to be most at risk. Such consumption becomes even more harmful when unsupervised by professionals. Further consideration should also be given to the importance of mind–body training and the development of a more compassionate attitude towards oneself, in order to avoid an unwanted objectification of the human body, excessive exercising, and other damaging behaviours. Such skills are often omitted from sports training, but their benefits have been well documented in martial arts and yoga, and might be applicable to other disciplines.

We hope that the research findings and suggestions discussed in this chapter can contribute to a more informed debate about the definition of 'good exercise habits' in terms of the health benefits of a range of different forms of exercise during exceptional circumstances, such as the COVID-19 pandemic.

References

1 Japanese Association of Occupational Therapists. *eSports Offer a New "Participation" Opportunity for People with Disabilities.* Japanese Association of Occupational Therapists, 2020. www.jaot.or.jp/en/

2 Ashcraft B. *Korean eSports Player Passes Away at 25 Years Old.* Kotaku, 2013. https://kotaku.com/korean-esports-player-passes-away-at-25-years-old-493447342

3   Shimbun A. Citizen's groups in Saitama are working to bring e-sports to senior citizens to prevent dementia and promote health, and to interact with people of all ages. Asahi Shimbun, 2020. www.saitama-np.co.jp/news/2020/07/26/10.html

4   Corazza O, Simonato P, Demetrovics Z et al. The emergence of Exercise Addiction, Body Dysmorphic Disorder, and other image-related psychopathological correlates in fitness settings: a cross sectional study. *PLoS ONE* 2019; 14: e0213060.

5   Terry A, Szabo A, Griffiths MD. The Exercise Addiction Inventory: a new brief screening tool. *Addict Res Theory* 2004; 12: 489–99.

6   Banz BC, Yip SW, Yau YH, Potenza MN. Behavioral addictions in addiction medicine: from mechanisms to practical considerations. *Prog Brain Res* 2016; 223: 311–28.

7   Fineberg NA, Demetrovics Z, Stein DJ et al. Manifesto for a European research network into problematic usage of the Internet. *Eur Neuropsychopharmacol* 2018; 28: 1232–46.

8   Lichtenstein MB, Griffiths MD, Hemmingsen SD, Støving RK. Exercise addiction in adolescents and emerging adults – validation of a youth version of the Exercise Addiction Inventory. *J Behav Addict* 2018; 7: 117–25.

9   Petry NM., Zajac K, Ginley MK. Behavioral addictions as mental disorders: to be or not to be? *Annu Rev Clin Psychol* 2018; 14: 399–423.

10 Shibata M, Burkauskas J, Dores AR et al. Exploring the relationship between mental well-being, exercise routines, and the intake of image and performance enhancing drugs during the coronavirus disease 2019 pandemic: a comparison across sport disciplines. *Front Psychol* 2021; 12: 689058.

11 Di Lodovico L, Poulnais S, Gorwood P. Which sports are more at risk of physical exercise addiction: a systematic review. *Addict Behav* 2019; 93: 257–62.

12 Trott M, Yang L, Jackson SE et al. Prevalence and correlates of exercise addiction in the presence vs. absence of indicated eating disorders. *Front Sports Act Living* 2020; 2: 84.

13 Neff KD. Self-compassion: an alternative conceptualization of a healthy attitude toward oneself. *Self Identity* 2003; 2: 85–101.

14 Maida D, Armstrong S. The classification of muscle dysmorphia. *Int J Men's Health* 2005; 4: 73–91.

15 Mosley PE. Bigorexia: bodybuilding and muscle dysmorphia. *Eur Eat Disord Rev* 2009; 17: 191–8.

16 Claudino JG, Gabbett TJ, Bourgeois F et al. CrossFit overview: systematic review and meta-analysis. *Sports Med Open* 2018; 4: 11.

17 Lichtenstein MB, Jensen TT. Exercise addiction in CrossFit: prevalence and psychometric properties of the Exercise Addiction Inventory. *Addict Behav Rep* 2016; 3: 33–7.

18 Hassmén P, Koivula N, Uutela A. Physical exercise and psychological well-being: a population study in Finland. *Prev Med* 2000; 30: 17–25.

19 Neff KD. The development and validation of a scale to measure self-compassion. *Self Identity* 2003; 2: 223–50.

20 Barczak N, Eklund RC. The moderating effect of self-compassion on relationships between performance and subsequent coping and motivation. *Int J Sport Exerc Psychol* 2020; 18: 256–68.

21 Phelps CL, Paniagua SM, Willcockson IU, Potter JS. The relationship between self-compassion and the risk for substance use disorder. *Drug Alcohol Depend* 2018; 183: 78–81.

22 Wisner M, Khoury B. Is self-compassion negatively associated with alcohol and marijuana-related problems via coping motives? *Addict Behav* 2020; 111: 106554.

23 Nakao M, Ohara C. The perspective of psychosomatic medicine on the effect of religion on the mind–body relationship in Japan. *J Relig Health* 2014; 53: 46–55.

24 Bond AR, Mason HF, Lemaster CM et al. Embodied health: the effects of a mind–body course for medical students. *Med Educ Online* 2013; 18: 1–8.

25 Fujiwara H, Ueno T, Yoshimura S et al. Martial arts "*Kendo*" and the motivation network during attention processing: an fMRI study. *Front Hum Neurosci* 2019; 13: 170.

26 Morisawa T, Watanabe M, Mori H et al. Can traditional breathing methods reduce stress? *Health* 2020; 12: 923–31.

27 Mooventhan A, Nivethitha L. Evidence based effects of yoga in neurological disorders. *J Clin Neurosci* 2017; 43: 61–7.

28 Hofmann SG, Andreoli G, Carpenter JK, Curtiss J. Effect of Hatha yoga on anxiety: a meta-analysis. *J Evid Based Med* 2016; 9: 116–24.

29 De Manincor M, Bensoussan A, Smith CA et al. Individualized yoga for reducing depression and anxiety, and improving well-being: a randomized controlled trial. *Depress Anxiety* 2016; 33: 816–28.

30 Falsafi N. A randomized controlled trial of mindfulness versus yoga: effects on depression and/or anxiety in college students. *J Am Psychiatr Nurses Assoc* 2016; 22: 483–97.

31 Suino N. Training the mind. In: *Budo Mind and Body: Training Secrets of the Japanese Martial Arts.* Shambhala Publications Inc., 2006: 29–40.

32 Nakamura S. *Zen Practice and Self-Control.* Komazawa University, 1995.

From Exercise to Addiction: An Introduction to the Phenomenon

The Ideal of the Perfect Body

Appearance Anxiety, Excessive Exercising, and Use of Image- and Performance-Enhancing Drugs

Artemisa Rocha Dores and Irene P. Carvalho

5.1 Body Image: Concept and Theoretical Frameworks

The concept of body image was initially coined by Schilder with reference to the mental representation that a person forms of their own body, including aspects such as shape, size, and weight [1]. In a more complete way, body image involves four fundamental dimensions: (i) a perceptual dimension (i.e., the way a person views their body, including an overall awareness of the body as a whole); (ii) a cognitive dimension (i.e., a person's thoughts and feelings about their body); (iii) an affective dimension (i.e., a person's feelings about how their body looks); and (iv) a behavioural dimension (i.e., what the person does about their perceived appearance) [2,3]. Based on the third dimension in this list, this subjective view of the body can be either positive or negative, depending on whether it is associated with satisfaction, acceptance, and comfort or with dissatisfaction, shame, and anxiety.

Schilder was the first researcher who sought to understand the experience of the body within a psychological and sociological framework. This perspective reflects the understanding that each person's perception is not limited to a cognitive construction, but is also the result of the attitudes of others, and of the interactions with others [1]. From this perspective, the body is a social phenomenon as well as a psychological construct. The English term 'body' is derived from an old Saxon word that means 'vessel', which can be viewed as a material container for the person, or for the person's mind. The focus on the body as a physical, inactive, or neutral carrier of the actual person – that is, as the biological machine for the mind – can be attributed to the legacy of René Descartes' (1596–1650) mind–body dualism. The Cartesian dualism emphasizes that thought is disembodied [4], and thus the body would be independent from thought, or from the mind. Yet the body can be subjectively experienced and invested in, and can be a representation or vehicle of the self [5] in terms of psychosomatic symptoms (defined by Edward Shorter as physical symptoms created by the mind without organic causes) or identities (e.g., healthy vs. unhealthy, normal vs. abnormal, beautiful vs. ugly) [6]. Furthermore, the notion that reality (including one's body) is socially constructed has long been recognized, dating back to the traditions of symbolic interactionism in sociology, or Bandura's social learning theory in psychology. From this perspective, the body as a social construction has implications for the meaning of 'correct' or 'ideal' bodies throughout time, a notion that is captured in Umberto Eco's works on the constantly changing concepts of beauty and ugliness as depicted in images and art throughout history [7,8]. For example, Foucault argued that the practice of freedom among the ancient Greeks and Romans involved an existence that had as its primary focus the body and its pleasures [9]. The early Christian culture required renunciation of the self (and of the body), whereas the eighteenth century demanded the constitution of a new self [10]. With the advent of today's consumer culture, which several authors have described as a culture of narcissism [11,12], the conception of the self 'places greater emphasis on appearance, display and the management of impressions' [11; p. 27] and 'the body is the passport to all that is good in life. Health, youth, beauty, sex, fitness are the positive attributes which body care can achieve and preserve' [11; p. 26]. In summary, the body, which has also been a focus of academic interest since the late 1980s [4], is no longer viewed, or experienced, as merely a 'biological vessel', but is now considered to be a psychological, social, cultural, and historical phenomenon.

Sociocultural theories of body image postulate that different societies have different conceptions of the ideal body shape, which are disseminated through various means, including family, peers, and the media. For example, aligning with *social learning models*, the *tripartite influence model of body image* posits that the three primary sources of influence and transmission of bodily ideals are one's parents, one's peers, and the media [13]. In an international study that surveyed 7,434 individuals from 10 different world regions about the body, significant cross-regional differences were found with regard to the ideal female figure and body dissatisfaction. For example, participants from low-socioeconomic-status sites preferred heavier bodies than did participants from high-socioeconomic-status sites in Malaysia and South Africa, but not in Austria. In addition, exposure to Western media predicted body weight ideals and also body dissatisfaction among women [14].

5.2 The Media and Self-Perception of Body Image

In Westernized cultures, people are constantly bombarded with advertisements containing messages that promote and reflect assumptions about the 'ideal' or 'desirable' body. Such messages simultaneously reinforce and perpetuate certain archetypes of beauty as a superior social value. This 'normalization' of bodies can even lead 'to changing the definition or the perception of what a "normal" body is', in the words of Georges Canguilhem, 'by means of the persuasion of advertising' [15; p. 247]. These messages become internalized, leading to the sense of a discrepancy between one's real body and the ideal body, generating dissatisfaction [16]. The distorted perception of body image is thus reinforced by the media because the point of reference that is used to judge attractiveness is unrealistic, and can lead to the perception of lack of attractiveness, body dissatisfaction, and even body image disorders.

The Internet, and especially social media networks, have contributed to an increase in this phenomenon [17,18]. Compared with traditional means of mass communication, the easy accessibility and permanent availability of smartphones and other devices, as well as the widespread and growing popularity of social media, mean that the latter have a much greater influence potential. Pervasive images can have a powerful impact on how the body is perceived and evaluated [18–21]. Several studies have suggested that active involvement in social networks can negatively influence body image, and appears to be associated with body dissatisfaction, eating disorders, use of image- and performance-enhancing drugs (IPEDs) such as anabolic steroids, and 'addiction' to physical exercise [22,23].

The influence of the Internet and other virtual networks operates in many of the same ways as do real-world social interactions, namely through brand and industry advertisements and via social interactions among users. The Internet additionally increases exposure through other means, such as depiction of the body in video games, for example, with images portraying the male body as unrealistically muscular [24]. In view of the widespread and growing use of the Internet, such trends have important implications for individuals' psychological well-being, calling for the need of a better understanding of these phenomena.

One example of the effects of industry advertisements is a recent trend called 'fitspiration' (a combination of the words 'fitness' and 'inspiration', often shortened to 'fitspo'), which promotes health content. Although originally aimed at encouraging healthier lifestyles, its content, targeted at aspects such as self-care, healthy diets, and fitness, often conveys distressing and potentially harmful messages related to body image and excessive exercising [23,25,26]. Social media might have contributed to this 'fitspirational' trend through the constant posting of photos and videos depicting 'perfect' bodies, and inspirational messages encouraging people to exercise.

In an intervention study, Prichard et al. looked at the effects of viewing Instagram inspirational images on body dissatisfaction, mood, and exercise among young women [27]. They also assessed whether engaging in exercise after exposure to inspirational images could mitigate any of the negative effects of exposure to such images. Body dissatisfaction and mood were assessed at baseline, after exposure to fitspiration or travel inspiration images, and after a 10-minute walk or quiet rest. The results showed that exposure to fitspiration images led to significantly higher levels of negative mood and body dissatisfaction, compared with exposure to travel images. Exposure to fitspiration images did not lead to an increase in actual exercising. Overall, negative mood and body dissatisfaction decreased after both exercise and quiet rest.

When using social networks and the Internet for social interactions, users publish photos of themselves (i.e., 'selfies') and view photos of others, with physical appearance being an important aspect of these activities. Users receive messages and comments about their bodies, and many of the photographs that are viewed or displayed are carefully selected and edited for a closer approximation of the images to the 'thin' or 'fit' inspiration. The potentially harmful effects of exposure to this type of images have been documented in several studies that examined their impact on quality of life and mental health [21,28]. For example, a study on the relationship between body image and the use of Facebook, conducted among a sample of more than 1,087 girls, showed that almost all (95.9%) of the participants had Internet access at home, and 75% of them had a Facebook profile and spent an average of 1.5 hours per day on it. Time spent on the Internet was significantly related to the internalization of the thin ideal, body vigilance, and the search for thinness. Facebook users also scored significantly higher than non-users on all measures of concern about body image. The researchers concluded that the Internet represents a powerful socio-cultural medium of relevance to the body image of adolescent girls [29].

In another study, conducted among women who used Facebook, those who spent time on Facebook reported a more negative mood than did those who spent time on the control website (an online fashion magazine website). Women who displayed a greater tendency to compare their appearance with that of others reported having more facial, hair-, and skin-related discrepancies after Facebook exposure than after exposure to the control website [30]. Thus it seems that social trends have developed which favour the comparison of one's own body with the ideals of appearance that are presented on social media platforms, as well as the internalization of these ideals, and the process of self-objectification [31]. When a person's physical appearance does not correspond to their internalized ideals, body dissatisfaction can develop.

5.3 Images of the Body in Modern Western Cultures

Body-related ideals that are commonly promoted in current Westernized cultures focus on thin bodies for girls and women (sometimes referred to as the thin, beautiful, or cultural ideal), and lean, muscular bodies for boys and men. The social stigma of obesity causes overweight people to be perceived as inadequate from childhood onwards [32]. The experience of bullying related to being overweight contributes to the development of negative body perceptions and body dissatisfaction. Even in adulthood, people with excessive body weight may have fewer opportunities in the labour market and experience discrimination in the workplace [33].

Consistent with these social values, there is a consensus that most men aspire to a mesomorphic body type, characterized by a medium build, well-developed chest, arm, and shoulder muscles, and a slim waist and hips, rather than an ectomorphic (thin) or endomorphic (fat) body type [34–36]. Having a flat, toned abdomen is seen by some as a symbol of status in its own right [37,38]. Being thin is seen as a status symbol that can be acquired independently of whether one possesses easily attainable material goods (e.g., technological equipment) [20]. Hall et al. have reported that men, like women, are becoming increasingly interested in their body image and are spending more money on beauty products and services, which they view as necessary for securing certain jobs and for career advancement [39].

Studies on the use of substances to increase the muscles have supported the idea that men feel under pressure to develop more muscular bodies, and that this pressure has increased in the twenty-first century. For instance, McCreary and Saucier carried out extensive research on men's motivation to develop muscular bodies [40]. They showed the importance of the muscular ideal for men, and the association between the desire to be more muscular, low self-esteem, depression, and psychological distress. Body image concerns were evident among both older and younger men, and participation in a weight loss programme was associated with a significant increase in confidence, self-esteem, and psychological well-being for those who lost weight [41]. Among women, concern about fat, diet, and being slim can even be considered as normative, given the strong messages conveyed in Western cultures that women's bodies should be completely under control, toned, and contained – an ideal that can only be achieved through diet or extreme exercise and weight training [42].

Susan Bordo is one of the authors who has studied the social meanings of different body phenotypes [42]. At the end of the twentieth century she identified an association between body appearance and the perception of positive or negative personal qualities, linked to low or high body weight, respectively. Such qualities included lack of willpower and personal inadequacy, as opposed to willpower, energy, control, and success. Among both men and women, excessive weight tends to be seen as physically unattractive and as associated with other negative characteristics. In general, being slender and thin is associated with happiness, success, youthfulness, and social acceptance, whereas excessive weight is linked to laziness, lack of willpower, and the perception of being out of control [20]. The famous phrase 'What is beautiful is good' encapsulates this association between beauty, character, and life outcomes that are more favourable to people who are perceived as attractive [43]. However, the majority of the population does not have naturally toned and slim bodies.

To achieve the desired 'perfect' body, there is a need for constant control and surveillance, whether through exercise, diet, or plastic surgery [42,44]. The idea of the female body as inherently imperfect and in need of reconstruction seems also to have created the need for this type of service, and in the 1990s there was an emphasis on body ornamentation and the remodelling of the female body [45].

Several studies have reported that the ideals of a muscular male body and a thin female beauty are associated with a range of psychological changes, including a distorted perception of body image [46], which can lead to the development of a mental disorder. Pressure to lose weight or gain muscle is often associated with body dissatisfaction and associated disturbances [47]. These body image disturbances have been studied in the scope of multifactorial theoretical models, such as those mentioned at the beginning of this chapter. Such theoretical models assume that a whole range of factors can be involved in the aetiology and maintenance of distress about body image, including psychological, social, cultural, biological, historical, and individual factors [48].

5.4 Distress About Body Image

Anxiety about one's appearance might culminate into body dysmorphic disorder (BDD) [49]. This disorder is characterized by extreme dissatisfaction with minor flaws in one's appearance, together with an irresistible urge to eliminate such flaws by various means, including compulsive exercise and compulsive use of muscle-enhancing substances [49].

BDD has been associated with clinical conditions, including obsessive-compulsive disorder, eating disorders, addictive behaviours, and, among men, muscle dysmorphia [49,50]. It is one of the most likely displayed mental disorders [49]. However, it is still an under-recognized and frequently under-diagnosed condition [51], despite its significant interference with different life domains, including social functioning [52,53]. The specific aetiology and pathophysiology of BDD within the spectrum of severe obsessive-compulsive behaviours are still under debate (e.g., [50]), and the number of studies on this subject has increased, highlighting its relevance.

5.5 Physical Exercise and Excessive Use

It is well documented that physical exercise decreases the incidence of heart disease, blood pressure, and diabetes [54], and the World Health Organization has recommended that, to protect heart function, adults aged 18–64 years should do 150 minutes of moderate-intensity aerobic physical activity every week [53]. In addition, regular exercise is beneficial for physical, psychological, and social well-being [55,56]. Educational and health institutions, together with the media, have increasingly promoted the beneficial effects of exercise and leanness over the years [57]. Perhaps as a consequence, there has been a growing acceptance, over time, of exercise as a fundamental part of a healthy lifestyle, and it has become an integral part of the daily routine or habits of people of all ages, playing a crucial role in health promotion and disease prevention [57,58].

Although health-related arguments are used to emphasize the importance of low body weight, historically thinness has not always been linked to health.

On the contrary, it was associated with diseases such as tuberculosis and HIV in the past. It was only at the end of the twentieth century and in the early years of this century that the belief that thinness is an indicator of good health became widespread [20]. Nevertheless, people's motives for engaging in physical exercise might not be directly related to health, even if benefits to health are an indirect consequence. For example, a study with 93 British employees about the reasons for exercising showed that the main motivating factor among the women who were interviewed was to improve muscle tone and lose weight, rather than to improve health or other reasons, such as the pleasure of exercising.

Weight loss is a more important motivator for women who exercise than for men, and women and gay men are more likely than heterosexual men to exercise to improve their overall appearance [20]. These results are consistent with the findings that Furnham and Greaves reported in the 1990s [59], and suggest that women's motives for exercising might differ from those of men. Nevertheless, although men are significantly less likely than women to be motivated to exercise to improve their appearance [60], a significant proportion of men do use exercise to try to change their appearance [61]. The authors suggest that, among men, the desire to be more muscular and toned has the potential to influence their health positively by encouraging involvement in exercise.

Weight training and sports that have the effect of increasing muscle mass are among the preferred activities for improving body image [61]. Thus exercise can be used to improve physical appearance, with the potential for positive effects on body image and self-esteem. However, the concept of exercise as a beauty treatment can lead to unrealistic expectations, which might result in the abandonment of exercising when those goals are not achieved. The competitive nature of sports environments can also alienate those whose bodies do not conform to the idealized image [62]. Research on the relationship between physical exercise and body image is still controversial. However, the sociocultural pressure on men and women of different ages to achieve the ideal body can lead to excessive involvement in this type of activity, which might result in the development of exercise dependence [63,64], especially in a culture where social criticism of this practice is low [65].

Engaging in excessive physical exercise can potentially be as dangerous to health as any other behavioural or substance addiction [66]. Different studies indicate the possible negative effects of excessive exercise, which range from psychological distress due to exercise deprivation as a result of injury to mental disorders such as anxiety and depression [49,55].

Exercise dependence, like other dependences, can be characterized by the need for ever increasing amounts of exercise, the presence of withdrawal symptoms (e.g., restlessness, mood change, relapse, personal conflict, frustration) when exercising is suspended, the use of exercise to regulate emotions, impaired family relationships, weight loss, and loss of control over exercising [57]. Characteristics such as salience, mood modification, tolerance, withdrawal symptoms, conflict, and relapse [67,68] have been used not only to define exercise dependence, but also to differentiate it from strong commitment to exercising [69]. However, the construct of exercise addiction (EA) remains controversial and is not included in the 11th revision of the *International Classification of Diseases (ICD-11)* [70] or the fifth edition of the *Diagnostic and Statistical Manual of Mental Disorders (DSM-5)* [52], pending further research.

5.6 Use of IPEDs

In addition to physical exercise, supplements and drugs that are marketed as able to improve a person's image and performance have also been used in their attempts to attain a 'perfect' body. Problematic exercising has been associated with an escalation in the consumption of IPEDs [71]. These substances, also known as 'lifestyle drugs', include anabolic steroids and other drugs that can be used to modify the functions of the body so as to enhance muscle development, reduce body fat, and promote weight loss [72].

Online and television advertisements may be contributing to, and exacerbating the use of these drugs through misleading marketing strategies that promise a rapid and safe change in appearance [71]. However, IPEDs may contain undisclosed ingredients that can have potentially damaging effects on users who are unaware of these risks.

In addition to medically supervised procedures, there has also been an increase in Do it yourself ('DIY') muscle enhancement procedures over the last 20 years. For example, in the early twentieth century, oils were developed for use in localized aesthetic treatment procedures such as wrinkle reduction [73]. They are now used as injectable products, and are widely available for sale on internet bodybuilding sites [20], despite documented evidence that they can cause complications such as stroke, pulmonary embolism, localized skin problems, nerve damage and cysts, and muscle damage, all of which can have serious long-term effects on health [74].

The use of anabolic steroids as an aid to body improvement is becoming increasingly prevalent [75]. Because of their widespread availability in gyms and sports clubs in a number of countries, it is not possible to accurately determine the extent of non-medical use of steroids [76,77]. Their earliest documented use for this purpose dates back to the 1950s, when they were associated with weightlifting [78]. Steroids enable the user to build muscle much faster than is possible through weight training alone, making them an attractive option, and they have been used by professional bodybuilders to increase muscle mass. More recent studies suggest that steroids are now being used by growing numbers of young people who have aesthetic concerns about a negative body image [76,77,79].

Most research on anabolic steroid use has focused on male samples, consistent with the notion that most users are men [75]. For example, Hall et al. have shown that increasing numbers of men are injecting synthol into their muscles to increase muscle size – a practice that carries health risks [80]. However, women's use of anabolic steroid drugs for bodybuilding purposes has increased during the last 20 years [81,82]. Social encouragement (especially from within the bodybuilding community) and the belief that it is impossible to achieve the desired body without steroids are cited as reasons for their increased use among women, despite the known harmful consequences. These include masculinizing effects (male baldness and deepening of the voice), the threat to reproductive health, and associated serious long-term risks such as kidney damage, liver damage, or the risk of transmission of bloodborne diseases as a result of sharing needles. Men have also reported experiencing severe side effects (e.g., liver damage, kidney damage, hypertension), but described them as minor irritations that were not a significant disincentive to using steroids [60]. They attributed the side effects to 'abuse' of these products – that is, to uninformed and excessive use – and believed that steroids used in moderation did not pose significant health risks. Some have compared their overuse to the overuse of other substances, such as alcohol and over-the-counter painkillers. They tended to believe that the information conveyed by health professionals was not credible because it was not linked to users' experiences. Instead, the most trusted sources of information on the safe use of steroids were books written by members of the bodybuilding community, websites run by steroid users, and word-of-mouth information from other users.

5.7 Practice Implications and Conclusions

This chapter has documented how societal pressure on body image can contribute to negative effects on the individual. Body image dissatisfaction has been associated with a number of different factors. Individual characteristics and predispositions interact with social, historical, and cultural norms. In view of the potential impact of societal pressure on physical and mental health, measures that can contribute to the protection of the most vulnerable individuals are urgently needed in terms of regulatory action, policy, and practice. For example, the Mental Health Foundation recommends the structured regulation of social media and advertising, greater exposure to a diversity of body types in the media, presence of clear systems, in social media companies, for reporting discrimination and stigma, and, as part of healthcare and public health action, inclusion of training of frontline practitioners to support those in crisis and in distress. In addition, there is a need to launch obesity campaigns that address the issue of education in schools, and develop students' media literacy [83]. Actions at the individual and community level are also suggested, as well as actions aimed at specific populations, including children, young people, those with long-term conditions and disabilities, people from different cultures and ethnic groups, and the lesbian, gay, bisexual, and transgender (LGBT) community.

Reflecting these calls for change, initiatives such as the Body Positive Movement and the Dove Self-Esteem Project have been promoting a more flexible body image for all, irrespective of age, gender, or race, including acceptance of body diversity (e.g., size diversity and body acceptance). Taken together, these measures can be part of a process of change that potentially leads to a more accepting and integrative view of diversity, and that contributes to a more positive body image and improved health.

References

1   Schilder P. *The Image and Appearance of the Human Body*. Kegan Paul, 1935.

2   Head H, Holmes G. *Les Sensations et el Córtex Cerebral [The Sensations and the Cerebral Cortex]*. Privat, 1973.

3   Schilder P. *A Imagem do Corpo. As Energias Construtivas da Psique [The Body Image. The Constructive Energies of the Psyche]*. Martins Fontes, 1980.

4   Fraser M, Greco M. Introduction. In: Fraser M, Greco M, eds. *The Body: A Reader*. Routledge, 2005: 26–41.

5   Turner B. *The Body and Society*. Sage, 1996.

6   Shorter E. *From Paralysis to Fatigue: A History of Psychosomatic Illness in the Modern Era*. Free Press, 1992.

7   Eco U. *Storia della Bruttezza [On Uglyness]*. RCS Libri S.p.A. Bompiani, 2007.

8   Eco U, de Michele G. *Storia della Bellezza [On Beauty]*. RCS Libri S.p.A. Bompiani, 2002.

9   Foucault M. *The Use of Pleasure: The History of Sexuality*, Vol. 2. Penguin, 1986.

10 Foucault M. Technologies of the self. In: Martin LM, Gutman H, Hutton PH, eds. *Technologies of the Self: A Seminar with Michel Foucault*. Tavistock, 1988: 16–49.

11 Featherstone M. The body in consumer culture. *Theory Cult Soc* 1982; 1: 18–33.

12 Lipovetsky G. *L'Ère du Vide [The Era of the Void]*. Gallimard, 1983.

13 van den Berg P, Thompson JK, Obremski-Brandon K, Coovert M. The Tripartite Influence model of body image and eating disturbance: a covariance structure modeling investigation testing the mediational role of appearance comparison. *J Psychosom Res* 2002; 53: 1007–20.

14 Swami V, Frederick DA, Aavik T et al. The attractive female body weight and female body dissatisfaction in 26 countries across 10 world regions: results of the International Body Project I. *Pers Soc Psychol Bull* 2010; 36: 309–25.

15 Canguilhem G. *The Normal and the Pathological*. Zone, 1989.

16　Behar AR. La construcción cultural del cuerpo: el paradigma de los trastornos de la conducta alimentaria [The cultural construction of the body: the paradigm of eating disorders]. *Rev Chil Neuro-Psiquiatr* 2010; 48: 319–34.

17　Burnette CB, Kwitowski MA, Mazzeo SE. "I don't need people to tell me I'm pretty on social media:" a qualitative study of social media and body image in early adolescent girls. *Body Image* 2017; 23: 114–25.

18　Fardouly J, Vartanian LR. Social media and body image concerns: current research and future directions. *Curr Opin Psychol* 2016; 9: 1–5.

19　Barry CT, Doucette H, Loflin DC, Rivera-Hudson N, Herrington L. "Let me take a selfie": associations between self-photography, narcissism, and self-esteem. *Psychol Pop Media Cult* 2017; 6: 48–60.

20　Grogan S. *Body Image: Understanding Body Dissatisfaction in Men, Women and Children*, 3rd ed. Routledge, 2016.

21　Mabe AG, Forney KJ, Keel PK. Do you "like" my photo? Facebook use maintains eating disorder risk. *Int J Eat Disord* 2014; 47: 516–23.

22　Dores AR, Carvalho IP, Burkauskas J et al. Exercise and use of enhancement drugs at the time of the COVID-19 pandemic: a multicultural study on coping strategies during self-isolation and related risks. *Front Psychiatry* 2021; 12: 648501.

23　Cataldo I, De Luca I, Giorgetti V et al. Fitspiration on social media: body-image and other psychopathological risks among young adults. A narrative review. *Emerg Trends Drugs Addict Health* 2021; 1: 100010.

24　Sylvia Z, King TK, Morse BJ. Virtual ideals: the effect of video game play on male body image. *Comput Hum Behav* 2014; 37: 183–8.

25　Tiggemann M, Zaccardo M. "Exercise to be fit, not skinny": the effect of fitspiration imagery on women's body image. *Body Image* 2015; 15: 61–7.

26　Tiggemann M, Zaccardo M. 'Strong is the new skinny': a content analysis of# fitspiration images on Instagram. *J Health Psychol* 2016; 23: 1003–11.

27　Prichard I, Kavanagh E, Mulgrew KE, Lim MS, Tiggemann M. The effect of Instagram #fitspiration images on young women's mood, body image, and exercise behaviour. *Body Image* 2020; 33: 1–6.

28　Ghaznavi J, Taylor LD. Bones, body parts, and sex appeal: an analysis of #thinspiration images on popular social media. *Body Image* 2015; 14: 54–61.

29　Tiggemann M, Slater A. NetGirls: the Internet, Facebook, and body image concern in adolescent girls. *Int J Eat Disord* 2013; 46: 630–3.

30　Fardouly J, Diedrichs PC, Vartanian LR, Halliwell E. Social comparisons on social media: the impact of Facebook on young women's body image concerns and mood. *Body Image* 2015; 13: 38–45.

31　Griffiths S, Murray SB, Krug I, McLean SA. The contribution of social media to body dissatisfaction, eating disorder symptoms, and anabolic steroid use among sexual minority men. *Cyberpsychol Behav Soc Netw* 2018; 21: 149–56.

32 Zamani Sani SH, Fathirezaie Z, Brand S et al. Physical activity and self-esteem: testing direct and indirect relationships associated with psychological and physical mechanisms. *Neuropsychiatr Dis Treat* 2016; 12: 2617–25.

33 Puhl RM, Latner JD. Stigma, obesity, and the health of the nation's children. *Psychol Bull* 2007; 133: 557–80.

34 Franko DL, Fuller-Tyszkiewicz M, Rodgers RF et al. Internalization as a mediator of the relationship between conformity to masculine norms and body image attitudes and behaviors among young men in Sweden, US, UK, and Australia. *Body Image* 2015;15: 54–60.

35 Grogan S, Richards H. Body image: focus groups with boys and men. *Men Masculinities* 2002; 4: 219–32.

36 Jankowski GS, Gough B, Fawkner H, Halliwell E, Diedrichs PC. Young men's minimisation of their body dissatisfaction. *Psychol Health* 2018; 33: 1343–63.

37 Pope HG Jr, Gruber AJ, Mangweth B et al. Body image perception among men in three countries. *Am J Psychiatry* 2000; 157: 1297–301.

38 Pope HG Jr, Phillips KA, Olivardia R. *The Adonis Complex: The Secret Crisis of Male Body Obsession*. The Free Press, 2000.

39 Hall M, Grogan S, Gough B, eds. *Chemically Modified Bodies: The Use of Diverse Substances for Appearance Enhancement*. Palgrave Macmillan, 2006.

40 McCreary DR, Saucier DM. Drive for muscularity, body comparison, and social physique anxiety in men and women. *Body Image* 2009; 6: 24–30.

41 Gough B, Seymour-Smith S, Matthews CR. Body dissatisfaction, appearance investment, and wellbeing: how older obese men orient to 'aesthetic health'. *Psychol Men Masc* 2016; 17: 84–91.

42 Bordo S. Feminism, Foucault and the politics of the body. In: Ramazanoglu C, ed. *Up Against Foucault: Explorations of Some Tensions Between Foucault and Feminism*. Routledge, 1993: 179–202.

43 Dion K, Berscheid E, Walster E. What is beautiful is good. *J Pers Soc Psychol* 1972; 24: 285–90.

44 Al-Raqqad HK, Al-Bourini ES, Al Talahin FM, Aranki RME. The impact of school bullying on students' academic achievement from teachers' point of view. *Int Educ Stud* 2017; 10: 44–50.

45 Darling-Wolf F. Texts in context: intertextuality, hybridity, and the negotiation of cultural identity in Japan. *J Commun Inq* 2000; 24: 134–55.

46 Kaewpradub N, Kiatrungrit K, Hongsanguansri S, Pavasuthipaisit C. Association among Internet usage, body image and eating behaviors of secondary school students. *Shanghai Arch Psychiatry* 2017;29: 208–17.

47 Duarte C, Pinto-Gouveia J. Body image flexibility mediates the effect of body image-related victimization experiences and shame on binge eating and weight. *Eat Behav* 2016; 23: 13–18.

48 Cash TF, Smolak L. Understanding body images: historical and contemporary perspectives. In: Cash TF, Smolak L, eds. *Body Image: A Handbook of Science, Practice, and Prevention.* Guilford Press, 2011: 3–11.

49 Corazza O, Simonato P, Demetrovics Z et al. The emergence of Exercise Addiction, Body Dysmorphic Disorder, and other image-related psychopathological correlates in fitness settings: a cross sectional study. *PLoS ONE* 2019; 14: e0213060.

50 Beucke JC, Sepulcre J, Buhlmann U et al. Degree connectivity in body dysmorphic disorder and relationships with obsessive and compulsive symptoms. *Eur Neuropsychopharmacol* 2016; 26: 1657–66.

51 Bewley A. The neglected psychological aspects of skin disease. *BMJ* 2017; 358: j3208.

52 American Psychiatric Association. *Diagnostic and Statistical Manual of Mental Disorders*, 5th ed. American Psychiatric Association, 2013.

53 World Health Organization. *WHO Guidelines on Physical Activity and Sedentary Behaviour.* World Health Organization, 2020. https://apps.who.int/iris/handle/10665/336656

54 Sanchis-Soler G, Tortosa-Martínez J, Manchado-Lopez C, Cortell-Tormo JM. The effects of stress on cardiovascular disease and Alzheimer's disease: physical exercise as a counteract measure. *Int Rev Neurobiol* 2020; 152: 157–93.

55 Lichtenstein MB, Nielsen RO, Gudex C, Hinze CJ, Jørgensen U. Exercise addiction is associated with emotional distress in injured and non-injured regular exercisers. *Addict Behav Rep* 2018; 8: 33–9.

56 Soundy A, Roskell C, Stubbs B, Probst M, Vancampfort D. Investigating the benefits of sport participation for individuals with schizophrenia: a systematic review. *Psychiatr Danub* 2015; 27: 2–13.

57 Berczik K, Szabó A, Griffiths MD et al. Exercise addiction: symptoms, diagnosis, epidemiology, and etiology. *Subst Use Misuse* 2012; 47: 403–17.

58 Ekelund U, Steene-Johannessen J, Brown WJ et al. Does physical activity attenuate, or even eliminate, the detrimental association of sitting time with mortality? A harmonised meta-analysis of data from more than 1 million men and women. *Lancet* 2016; 388: 1302–10.

59 Furnham A, Greaves N. Gender and locus of control correlates of body image dissatisfaction. *Eur J Pers* 1994; 8: 183–200.

60 Grogan S, Conner M, Smithson H. Sexuality and exercise motivations: are gay men and heterosexual women most likely to be motivated by concern about weight and appearance? *Sex Roles* 2006; 55: 567–72.

61 Kyrejto JW, Mosewich AD, Kowalski KC, Mack DE, Crocker PRE. Men's and women's drive for muscularity: gender differences and cognitive and behavioral correlates. *Int J Sport Exerc Psychol* 2008; 6: 69–84.

62 Mutrie N, Choi PYL. III. Is 'fit' a feminist issue? Dilemmas for exercise psychology. *Fem Psychol* 2000; 10: 544–51.

63 Ginis KAG, Bassett, RL. Exercise: effects on body image. In: Cash T, ed. *Encyclopedia of Body Image and Human Appearance.* Academic Press, 2012: 412–17.

64 Mooney R, Simonato P, Ruparelia R et al. The use of supplements and performance and image enhancing drugs in fitness settings: an exploratory cross-sectional investigation in the United Kingdom. *Hum Psychopharmacol* 2017; 32. e2619.

65 Laus MF, Costa TMB, Almeida SS. Body image dissatisfaction and aesthetic exercise in adolescents: are they related? *Estud Psicol* 2013; 18: 63–171.

66 de Coverley Veale DM. Exercise dependence. *Br J Addict* 1987; 82: 735–40.

67 Griffiths MD. Behavioural addiction: an issue for everybody? *J Workplace Learn* 1996; 8: 19–25.

68 Griffiths MD. Exercise addiction: a case study. *Addict Res* 1997; 5: 161–8.

69 Cockerill IM, Riddington ME. Exercise dependence and associated disorders: a review. *Couns Psychol Q* 1996; 9: 119–29.

70 World Health Organization. *ICD-11 for Mortality and Morbidity Statistics.* World Health Organization, 2019.

71 Corazza O, Bersani FS, Brunoro R et al. The diffusion of performance and image-enhancing drugs (PIEDs) on the Internet: the abuse of the cognitive enhancer piracetam. *Subst Use Misuse* 2014; 49: 1849–56.

72 Bates G, McVeigh J. *Image and Performance Enhancing Drugs: 2015 Survey Results.* Centre for Public Health, Liverpool John Moores University, 2016. www.ipedinfo .co.uk/resources/downloads/2015%20National%20IPED%20Info%20Survey% 20report.pdf

73 Di Benedetto G, Pierangeli M, Scalise A, Bertani A. Paraffin oil injection in the body: an obsolete and destructive procedure. *Ann Plast Surg* 2002; 49: 391–6.

74 Banke IJ, Prodinger PM, Waldt S et al. Irreversible muscle damage in bodybuilding due to long-term intramuscular oil injection. *Int J Sports Med* 2012; 33: 829–34.

75 Smith D, Rutty MC, Olrich TW. Muscle dysmorphia and anabolic-androgenic steroid use. In: Hall M, Grogan S, Gough B, eds. *Chemically Modified Bodies: The Use of Diverse Substances for Appearance Enhancement.* Palgrave Macmillan, 2016: 31–50.

76 Hildebrandt T, Alfano L. Drug use, appearance- and performance-enhancing. In: Cash T, ed. *Encyclopedia of Body Image and Human Appearance.* Academic Press, 2012: 392–8.

77 Sagoe D, Andreassen CS, Pallesen S. The aetiology and trajectory of anabolic–androgenic steroid use initiation: a systematic review and synthesis of qualitative research. *Subst Abuse Treat Prev Policy* 2014; 9: 27.

78 Strauss RH, Yesalis CE. Anabolic steroids in the athlete. *Annu Rev Med* 1991; 42: 449–57.

79 Grogan S, Shepherd S, Evans R, Wright S, Hunter G. Experiences of anabolic steroid use: in-depth interviews with men and women body builders. *J Health Psychol* 2006; 11: 845–56.

80 Hall M, Grogan S, Gough B. Bodybuilders' accounts of synthol use: the construction of lay expertise. In: Hall M, Grogan S, Gough B, eds. *Chemically Modified Bodies: The Use of Diverse Substances for Appearance Enhancement.* Palgrave Macmillan, 2016: 127–45.

81 Eisenberg ME, Wall M, Neumark-Sztainer D. Muscle-enhancing behaviors among adolescent girls and boys. *Pediatrics* 2012; 130: 1019–26.

82 O'Dea J, Cinelli RL. Use of drugs to change appearance in girls and female adolescents. In: Hall M, Grogan S, Gough B, eds. *Chemically Modified Bodies: The Use of Diverse Substances for Appearance Enhancement.* Palgrave Macmillan, 2016: 51–76.

83 Mental Health Foundation. *Body Image: How We Think and Feel About Our Bodies.* Mental Health Foundation, 2019. www.mentalhealth.org.uk/publications/body-image-report.

From Exercise to Addiction: An Introduction to the Phenomenon

Exercise, Fitspiration, and the Role of Social Media

Ilaria De Luca, Dorotea Cicconcelli,
Valentina Giorgetti, and Ornella Corazza

6.1 Introduction

In our consumerist and hyper-connected society, fitness goals and beauty ideals are promoted and amplified by the now very widespread use of the Internet and social networking sites, which are fast becoming the main source of information and inspiration, especially for teenagers and young adults [1,2]. Social networks allow users to access and share a large amount of information, as well as to interact and communicate with other individuals online [3,4]. On these peer-generated platforms, everyone can publish or be exposed to advice, suggestions, and recommendations, without the need for any expertise.

In recent years, beauty ideals seem to have been undergoing a slight change, with the introduction of a more athletic body ideal that is widespread under the hashtag #fitspiration, or its short form #fitspo [5,6]. The concept of 'fitspiration' – a combination of the words 'fitness' and 'inspiration' – encourages people to engage in physical activity and adopt a healthy lifestyle [7]. Currently on Instagram there are 18.5 million posts with the hashtag #fitspiration [8]. Among active users on Instagram, it is possible to distinguish between Instagrammers and followers. People who systematically share images, texts, or fitspiration videos are defined as 'fitstagrammers'. They inspire followers to enhance their well-being through physical activity, sharing images and information about their meals and their fitness routines, and showing physical changes by posting 'before' and 'after' photos

[9,10]. Female fitspiration subjects are toned but thin, whereas male models typically adhere to a muscular or hyper muscular body shape [11,12]. The constant focus on appearance, in association with the uncontrolled promotion of healthy food and fitness activity, may contribute to portraying an unrealistic ideal of the body, with potential negative consequences. Social media are used by all age groups, but the category of young adults (aged 20–24 years) is most frequently involved [2]. Information about health, lifestyle, and fitness is among the most researched online content [1], and seems to increase body image dissatisfaction not only in adolescents and young adults but also in pre-teenage girls (aged 11–12 years) [13]. Exposure to fitspiration's themes and content has been linked to negative mood, appearance anxiety, low self-esteem, and body image concerns such as body dysmorphic disorder (BDD) and muscle dysmorphia (MD). In severe cases, it can facilitate or maintain eating disorders, compulsive exercise, and the misuse of image- and performance-enhancing drugs (IPEDs) [14–17]. The latter include a wide range of products that are advertised online as a natural and safe aid to improving muscularity and appearance, and which can be associated with side effects as well as with doping and addiction phenomena [18].

This chapter analyses the phenomenon of fitspiration on social networks, focusing on potential physical and psychological risks. Although the fitspiration trend seems to promote healthy lifestyles, the majority of the content reflects unhealthy behaviours and misleading information. Fitness and nutritional goals are mostly associated with visual appearance, promoting potentially dangerous behaviours [19].

6.2 Typical Fitspiration Themes and Content

Blackstone and Herrmann observed that 80.8% of the posts which they analysed on the support pages of Facebook fitness groups were characterized by 'before' and 'after' photos, mainly focused on users' bodies; men's bodies were shown as well developed and muscular, whereas women's bodies were usually thin and athletic [19]. The majority of fitspiration images on Instagram depict people (63.7%), predominantly women (67.3%), in posed shots [6,19]. Only 2.8% of the images promote the benefits of exercise or convey positive body messages [19]. This is consistent with evidence which suggests that, among social media users, exercise is often driven by appearance-related rather than health-related goals [20]. A literature review identified eight main types of fitspiration content that may be associated with psychopathological risks (see Table 6.1) [21].

Table 6.1 Different types of fitspiration content that may be associated with psychopathological risks [21]

1 Body objectification	Attention is given to specific body parts rather than to the body as a whole; the face is often omitted from the picture
2 Physical appearance prioritized over health and well-being	Fitness is viewed as a means to look good and attain unrealistic beauty ideals, rather than as a way to improve health
3 Self-worth measured in centimetres	Fat loss is considered to be the result of personal success, and feelings of inadequacy are experienced when the expected shape-related goals are not achieved
4 Obsessive control of eating habits	Calorie tracking, monitoring of food, dietary restrictions, and intermittent fasting are suggested
5 Exposure to unsupervised supplement intake	Use of dietary supplements without medical supervision is often promoted
6 Pain as pleasure	Pain is viewed as a source of motivation, satisfaction, and pleasure
7 Physical and mental burnout	Users are encouraged to push their bodies to the limit and to keep going 'unless you puke, faint, or die'
8 Social isolation	Feelings of exclusion and being a misfit are observed among participants who consider themselves slightly overweight

6.2.1 Body Objectification

Fitspiration content, especially on Instagram and other image-based social networks, often tends to highlight only appealing body parts, such as arms, buttocks, legs, chest, or abdomen, omitting the face from the picture [6,12, 22]. The tendency to feel their own body from an objectified perspective may induce users to become less sensitive to pain [22,23], with important consequences for sports practice and exercise, in which sensitivity to pain and responses to bodily cues are fundamental to improving performance and avoiding injuries [22].

6.2.2 Physical Appearance Prioritized Over Health and Well-Being

In most cases, exercising is encouraged in order to achieve appearance-related goals, and the emphasis is on aesthetic perfection rather than body functionality [12,23,24]. Fitness is rarely internalized as a healthy and functional state, but rather it is viewed as a means to get in shape, look good, and attain a beauty ideal [10,14, 20].

6.2.3 Self-Worth Measured in Centimetres

Great attention is given to measurements of body parts, such as waist, stomach, thighs, upper arms, wrists, and neck, in order to check progress [19]. To achieve fat loss and muscle gain, individuals are motivated to eat healthily and exercise much more for the look than for health reasons [19,22].

6.2.4 Obsessive Control of Eating Habits

To achieve fast and visible results, fitspiration posts suggest that users should adopt dietary restrictions such as intermittent fasting, calorie restriction, or complete avoidance of certain types of food. Challenges are often promoted (e.g., '30 days sugar-free' or '7 days carbo-free'), but without any nutritional expertise or medical supervision [4,19].

6.2.5 Exposure to Unsupervised Supplement Intake

Through social networking sites, influencers promote the consumption of weight loss products and dietary supplements, including IPEDs [10]. Supplements include proteins, vitamins, amino acids, caffeine, mineral salts, and diuretic teas, and they are mainly promoted with misleading information and purchased online without medical supervision [24].

6.2.6 Pain as Pleasure

Pain is considered to be a drive to succeed, and thus the experience of pain is turned into a source of motivation, satisfaction, and pleasure. Captions such as 'Strength and discipline become my weapon, then pain and agony become my pleasure' and 'Suffer the pain of discipline or suffer the pain of regret' are used to turn physical and mental discomfort into a positive feeling, motivating users to push their bodies to the limit [4].

6.2.7 Physical and Mental Burnout

Fitspiration posts frequently contain messages of guilt about body weight and body shape [24,25]. Failure is considered to be a choice, and admitting to failure is seen as a sign of weakness and laziness [20,22]. Such messages may lead users to engage in pathological behaviours, such as over-training [4].

6.2.8 Social Isolation

Through social networking sites, fitspiration users can find people online who are facing the same challenges and difficulties in reaching their desired goal.

When the community becomes exclusive, this creates a sense of superiority among those who are part of it, with hostility towards those who are not. Criticism is considered to be a form of jealousy, and outsiders are defined as 'haters' [22]. As a result, individuals who consider themselves overweight may experience feelings of loneliness and exclusion.

6.3 Exercise Addiction and Other Psychopathological Risks of Fitspiration

As has been increasingly documented in the literature, fitspiration posts may promote harmful messages that can have negative consequences. A recent study reported that young women with low self-esteem, obsessive traits, and perfectionism are the most typical users, who interact with social media platforms to gain a sense of greater personal security and endorsement [10]. This can lead to body image distortion and both primary and secondary exercise addiction (EA) [7,25,26].

6.3.1 Body Image Disorders

The common link between fitspiration and psychopathological disorders is the importance of appearance, which has been demonstrated to be the main goal of fitspiration messages and advice [14, 20]. Qualitative analysis and experimental studies have reported that fitspiration exposure increases short-term negative mood and significantly decreases self-esteem [7,12,17,27]. These feelings may lead to harmful beliefs about one's own body [12,27,28]. Body dissatisfaction, defined as the negative subjective evaluation of one's own body, is associated with a wide range of psychopathological states and behaviours [29], such as depression [30], anxiety [31], and poor life quality [32]. Research has mainly focused on women, tending to assume that men are generally more satisfied with their bodies. However, it has been observed that men also experience body disturbances, although these are mostly related to the desire for muscularity. Women tend to show more dissatisfaction with a particular part of their body, such as hips or thighs, whereas men mainly focus on the upper torso or biceps [33,34]. Body dissatisfaction has also been observed in transgender and gender non-conforming (TGNC) individuals, who are more likely to self-prescribe and self-administer hormones (androgens or oestrogens) bought online without a medical consultation [35]. A preoccupation with body image and physical appearance is also the core feature of BDD and MD [36]. BDD is characterized by excessive preoccupation with imagined or slight physical defects in appearance, which can lead to clinically significant distress [37]. This preoccupation is associated with other psychological symptoms, such as low self-esteem, feelings of shame, depressive symptoms, anxiety, and guilt [38], especially in fitness settings [16]. The diagnostic criteria for MD, considered to be a subgroup of BDD in the fifth edition of the *Diagnostic and Statistical Manual of Mental Disorders (DSM-V)*, appear to overlap with the main themes promoted by fitspiration, such as preoccupation with one's appearance (characterized by the belief that one's body is not sufficiently lean and muscular) and an intense drive for muscularity (which may lead to long hours of lifting weights, excessive attention to diet, and use of supplements) [36].

6.3.2 Primary and Secondary Exercise Addiction

Some influencers motivate viewers to engage in extreme forms of exercise [4]. Messages such as 'Unless you puke, faint, or die, keep going' may encourage an excessive and compulsive form of workout, resulting in pathological behaviour [39–42]. It is possible to distinguish between primary and secondary EA. Primary EA occurs in the absence of an eating disorder, and weight loss is secondary to the goal of improving physical performance [43]. According to the Veale classification criteria for EA, exercise may become stereotyped and be associated with withdrawal symptoms such as mood swings, irritability, and insomnia. Individuals who are interested in fitspiration content on social media commonly show an obsessive training pattern that may cause physical problems (e.g., fatigue, recurrent injuries) and psychological distress (e.g., social withdrawal, depression, anxiety) [3,44,45].

Secondary EA can present as a combination of compulsive exercise and disordered eating, defining a secondary EA. Turner and Lefevre found a significant relationship between higher rates of Instagram use and a tendency to develop an obsession with eating healthy food (also known as orthorexia) that may lead to extreme diets or malnutrition, with consequent impairment of daily functioning [46,47]. Influencers promote unhealthy behaviours for achieving weight loss, such as restrictive food intake, calorie tracking, long fasts, and excessive body checking, which induces feelings of guilt about food intake [7,27]. It has been reported that women who posted fitspiration images had higher scores for disordered eating, drive for muscularity, and compulsive exercise compared with women who posted travel photos [45]. Compulsive exercise and appearance-related anxiety have been identified in various fitness settings [16], and can also be specifically associated with the use of IPEDs and fitness supplements [16,24,42]. Drug supplementation, which was initially mainly widespread among male bodybuilders, is now also increasing in the fitness community, particularly among women [48]. Influencers have become part of a new 'self-help culture' in which they advertise these drug supplements and discuss their experiences without having any particular expertise in the subject [48]. Recent reports have shown that these products may contain unsafe ingredients (e.g., heavy metals, hormones, illegal drugs), and that a number of unwanted side effects have been associated with the use of supplements (e.g., irritation, tachycardia, insomnia, mood fluctuations, diarrhoea, changes in libido). These negative effects are still rarely discussed [16,49], while supplement intake is perceived to be safe and indeed essential if one is to develop a fit and toned body [16].

6.4 Conclusion

Social networks have a crucial role in defining beauty standards and sharing new trends and ideas. This chapter has shown how the emphasis on well-being, having a fit body, and healthy lifestyle has made potentially pathological behaviours, such as dietary restriction, substance misuse, and overexercising, socially acceptable. Physical and mental distress are justified in the pursuit of the desired body, and feelings of weakness and worthlessness are common among fitspiration users. The social distancing that was necessary to curb the spread of COVID-19 during the pandemic strengthened the role of social networking sites and online communities, which became the main source of information and means of social connection, posing unprecedented challenges to public and mental health. In an ever-changing society, researchers and clinicians need to be able to detect and understand the potentially harmful effects of social network content, as addictive behaviours, body image disturbances, and substance misuse have a broad spectrum of severity, and exposure to such content may trigger the onset of psychiatric disease or worsen its symptoms [15].

The fitspiration trend could potentially be a useful tool for promoting a healthy lifestyle, by emphasizing the positive aspects of controlled exercise and healthy nutrition. However, more realistic and positive messages, which aim to reduce body dissatisfaction and psychological distress and to enhance self-esteem, should be encouraged.

References

1   Vaterlaus JM, Patten EV, Roche C, Young JA. #Gettinghealthy: the perceived influence of social media on young adult health behaviors. *Comput Human Behav* 2015; 45: 151–7.

2   Pew Research Center. *Social Media Fact Sheet*. Pew Research Center, 2018. www .pewresearch.org/internet/fact-sheet/social-media/

3   Holland G, Tiggemann M. A systematic review of the impact of the use of social networking sites on body image and disordered eating outcomes. *Body Image* 2016; 17: 100–10.

4   Ratwatte P, Mattacola E. An exploration of 'fitspiration' content on YouTube and its impacts on consumers. *J Health Psychol* 2021; 26: 935–46.

5   Tiggemann M. Sociocultural perspectives on body image. In: Cash T, ed. *Encyclopedia of Body Image and Human Appearance*. Academic Press, 2012: 758–65.

6   Tiggemann M, Zaccardo M. 'Strong is the new skinny': a content analysis of #fitspiration images on Instagram. *J Health Psychol* 2018; 23: 1003–11.

7   Tiggemann M, Zaccardo M. "Exercise to be fit, not skinny": the effect of fitspiration imagery on women's body image. *Body Image* 2015; 15: 61–7.

8   Instagram.com. *#fitspiration.* www.instagram.com/explore/tags/fitspiration/ (accessed 20 May 2020).

9   DiBisceglie S, Arigo D. Perceptions of #fitspiration activity on Instagram: patterns of use, response, and preferences among fitstagrammers and followers. *J Health Psychol* 2021; 26: 1233–42.

10   Pilgrim K, Bohnet-Joschko S. Selling health and happiness how influencers communicate on Instagram about dieting and exercise: mixed methods research. *BMC Public Health* 2019; 19: 1054.

11   Tiggemann M, Martins Y, Kirkbride A. Oh to be lean and muscular: body image ideals in gay and heterosexual men. *Psychol Men Masc* 2007; 8: 15–24.

12   Carrotte ER, Prichard I, Lim MSC. "Fitspiration" on social media: a content analysis of gendered images. *J Med Internet Res* 2017; 19: e95.

13   Tiggemann M, Slater A. NetTweens: the Internet and body image concerns in preteenage girls. *J Early Adolesc* 2014; 34: 606–20.

14   Simpson CC, Mazzeo SE. Skinny is not enough: a content analysis of fitspiration on Pinterest. *Health Commun* 2017; 32: 560–7.

15   Griffiths S, Castle D, Cunningham M et al. How does exposure to thinspiration and fitspiration relate to symptom severity among individuals with eating disorders? Evaluation of a proposed model. *Body Image* 2018; 27: 187–95.

16   Corazza O, Simonato P, Demetrovics Z et al. The emergence of Exercise Addiction, Body Dysmorphic Disorder, and other image-related psychopathological correlates in fitness settings: a cross sectional study. *PLoS ONE* 2019; 14: e0213060.

17   Prichard I, Kavanagh E, Mulgrew KE, Lim MS, Tiggemann M. The effect of Instagram #fitspiration images on young women's mood, body image, and exercise behaviour. *Body Image* 2020; 33: 1–6.

18   Corazza O, Bersani, FS, Brunoro, R et al. The diffusion of performance and image-enhancing drugs (PIEDs) on the Internet: the abuse of the cognitive enhancer piracetam. *Subst Use Misuse* 2014; 49: 1849–56.

19   Blackstone SR, Herrmann LK. Extreme body messages: themes from Facebook posts in extreme fitness and nutrition online support groups. *mHealth* 2018; 4: 33.

20   Raggatt M, Wright CJ, Carrotte E et al. "I aspire to look and feel healthy like the posts convey": engagement with fitness inspiration on social media and perceptions of its influence on health and wellbeing. *BMC Public Health* 2018; 18: 1002.

21   Cataldo I, De Luca I, Giorgetti V et al. Fitspiration on social media: body-image and other psychopathological risks among young adults. A narrative review. *Emerg Trends Drugs Addict Health* 2021; 1: 100010.

22 Deighton-Smith N, Bell BT. Objectifying fitness: a content and thematic analysis of #fitspiration images on social media. *Psychol Pop Media Cult* 2018; 7: 467–83.

23 Loughnan S, Haslam N, Murnane T et al. Objectification leads to depersonalization: the denial of mind and moral concern to objectified others. *Eur J Soc Psychol* 2010; 40: 709–17.

24 Mooney R, Simonato P, Ruparelia R et al. The use of supplements and performance and image enhancing drugs in fitness settings: an exploratory cross-sectional investigation in the United Kingdom. *Hum Psychopharmacol* 2017; 32: e2619.

25 Alberga AS, Withnell SJ, von Ranson KM. Fitspiration and thinspiration: a comparison across three social networking sites. *J Eat Disord* 2018; 6: 39.

26 Boepple L, Thompson JK. An exploration of appearance and health messages present in pregnancy magazines. *J Health Psychol* 2017; 22: 1862–8.

27 Easton S, Morton K, Tappy Z, Francis D, Dennison L. Young people's experiences of viewing the fitspiration social media trend: qualitative study. *J Med Internet Res* 2018; 20: e219.

28 Rosen JC. Body image disorder: definition, development, and contribution to eating disorders. In: Crowther JH, Tennenbaum DL, Hobfoll SE, Stephens MA, eds. *The Etiology of Bulimia: The Individual and Familial Context.* Hemisphere Publishing Corporation, 2013: 157–77.

29 Puhl RM, Heuer CA. Obesity stigma: important considerations for public health. *Am J Public Health* 2010; 100: 1019–28.

30 Stice E, Telch CF, Rizvi SL. Development and validation of the Eating Disorder Diagnostic Scale: a brief self-report measure of anorexia, bulimia, and binge-eating disorder. *Psychol Assess* 2000; 12: 123–31.

31 Bennett K, Stevens R. Weight anxiety in older women. *Eur Eat Disord Rev* 1996; 4: 32–9.

32 Ganem PA, de Heer H, Morera OF. Does body dissatisfaction predict mental health outcomes in a sample of predominantly Hispanic college students? *Pers Individ Differ* 2009; 46: 557–61.

33 Olivardia R, Pope HG Jr, Borowiecki JJ III, Cohane GH. Biceps and body image: the relationship between muscularity and self-esteem, depression, and eating disorder symptoms. *Psychol Men Masc* 2004; 5: 112–20.

34 Bassett-Gunter R, McEwan D, Kamarhie A. Physical activity and body image among men and boys: a meta-analysis. *Body Image* 2017; 22: 114–28.

35 Metastasio A, Negri A, Martinotti G, Corazza O. Transitioning bodies. The case of self-prescribing sexual hormones in gender affirmation in individuals attending psychiatric services. *Brain Sci* 2018; 8: 88.

36 Cuzzolaro M. Body dysmorphic disorder and muscle dysmorphia. In: Cuzzolaro M, Fassino S, eds. *Body Image, Eating, and Weight: A Guide to Assessment, Treatment, and Prevention.* Springer, 2018: 67–84.

37 American Psychiatric Association. *Diagnostic and Statistical Manual of Mental Disorders*, 5th ed. American Psychiatric Association, 2013.

38 Weingarden H, Renshaw KD, Tangney JP, Wilhelm S. Development and validation of the Body-Focused Shame and Guilt scale. *J Obsessive Compuls Relat Disord* 2016; 8: 9–20.

39 Freimuth M, Moniz S, Kim SR. Clarifying exercise addiction: differential diagnosis, co-occurring disorders, and phases of addiction. *Int J Environ Res Public Health* 2011; 8: 4069–81.

40 Berczik K, Szabó A, Griffiths MD et al. Exercise addiction: symptoms, diagnosis, epidemiology, and etiology. *Subst Use Misuse* 2012; 47: 403–17.

41 Landolfi E. Exercise addiction. *Sports Med* 2013; 43: 111–19.

42 De Luca I, Simonato P, Mooney R, Bersani G, Corazza O, Can exercise be an addiction? The evolution of 'fitspiration' in society. *Res Adv Psychiatry* 2017; 4: 27–34.

43 De Coverley Veale DM. Exercise addiction. *Br J Addict* 1987; 82: 735–40.

44 Veale D. Does primary exercise dependence really exist? In: Annett J, Cripps B, Steinberg H, eds. *Exercise Addiction: Motivation for Participation in Sport and Exercise*. British Psychological Society, 1995: 71–5.

45 Holland G, Tiggemann M. "Strong beats skinny every time": disordered eating and compulsive exercise in women who post fitspiration on Instagram. *Int J Eat Disord* 2017; 50: 76–9.

46 Bratman S. The health food eating disorder. *Yoga J* 1997; 8: 42–50.

47 Turner PG, Lefevre CE. Instagram use is linked to increased symptoms of orthorexia nervosa. *Eat Weight Disord* 2017; 22: 277–84.

48 Andreasson J, Johansson T. (Un)Becoming a fitness doper: negotiating the meaning of illicit drug use in a gym and fitness context. *J Sport Soc Issues* 2020; 44: 93–109.

49 Martínez-Sanz JM, Sospedra I, Ortiz CM et al. Intended or unintended doping? A review of the presence of doping substances in dietary supplements used in sports. *Nutrients* 2017; 9: 1093.

Eating Disorders and Over-Exercise

Charlotte Taylor, Kate Brown, and Konstantinos Ioannidis

7.1 Introduction

Eating disorders are a globally widespread problem with concerning implications for public health, and they represent an important health burden for societies worldwide [1,2]. They have the highest morbidity and mortality of all mental illnesses [3], and a significant lifetime prevalence, of around 1.2–2.4% for anorexia nervosa and around 1.2–2.3% for bulimia nervosa, depending on the diagnostic criteria used and the population under study [4]. In the literature the reported incidence of eating disorders varies, being higher in studies that used community samples than in those that focused on treatment-seeking individuals. In these disorders, compulsions can be manifested in the form of extreme dietary restriction and over-exercise [5]. It has been argued that clinicians and researchers working with people with eating disorders can benefit from prioritizing assessments that capture the compulsive qualities of exercise, which are essential for understanding the clinical profile of the individual [6] and contributing to a more accurate and detailed psychological formulation.

7.2 Exercise and Eating Disorders

Dysfunctional exercise (a term used here to encompass compulsive, excessive, 'obligatory' exercise, or over-exercise) is one of the most challenging disordered eating behaviours. It can also have many catastrophic consequences, and is a driver of medical morbidity. Dysfunctional exercise often develops after the onset of an eating disorder, acts as a key maintaining factor, and is one of the longer-term symptoms, taking longer to resolve [7]. In addition to causing precipitous weight loss, dysfunctional exercise in eating disorders leads to repetitive strain injuries (e.g., stress fractures, tendonitis, muscle tears), muscle imbalance, and related pain, with associated biomechanical changes in muscle and altered muscle function, heart abnormalities (e.g., life-threatening bradycardia), and rhabdomyolysis, among other medical complications [8,9]. Bone fractures are common, especially when dysfunctional exercise is coupled with osteoporosis (a common presentation in chronic and enduring anorexia nervosa), and these are caused by activity-related injuries. Excessive exercise in the context of eating disorders appears to occur predominantly among girls and women, in whom it has well-documented effects that include infertility, sleep disturbance, and abnormal energy levels [10]. Research on the effects of excessive exercise in boys and men is sparse, but appears to focus mainly on the psychological effects, such as muscle dysmorphia and rumination [11]. Bulimia nervosa cohorts are often associated with sport injuries; the individual is unable to stop exercising, resulting in an increased incidence of injury and the onset of chronic pain. Excessive exercise is seen in up to 80% of anorexia nervosa cohorts [12)]. In a 15-year prospective study of individuals with anorexia nervosa, compulsive excessive exercise at the time of discharge from hospital was identified as one of the most significant predictors of poor long-term treatment outcomes and early time to relapse [13].

Excessive exercise among individuals with eating disorders is not a uniquely Western phenomenon [14], although research suggests that it tends to be most prevalent in Western countries [15], especially among competitive occupations that focus on appearance, such as modelling and dance [16,17]. The competitive nature of the activity was found to have a mediating effect, and this has also been reported in other sporting industries where competition leads to over-exercising [18]. *Relative energy deficiency in sport (REDS)* is a recognized syndrome in which athletes, influenced by the perception that thinness and leanness can enhance athletic performance, alter both their training schedules and their nutritional intake to achieve this. However, these desired outcomes are not achieved, and the altered behaviours can lead to long-term complications and subsequent detrimental effects on both health and athletic performance [19].

Evolutionary theory suggests that once an individual's body weight falls below a certain value, a primal activation occurs whereby they begin to exhibit a fight or flight response, and the parasympathetic nervous system is unable to function due to the continual anticipation of threat and the need to survive and escape [20]. This theory suggests that weight loss does not reflect a need to be thin, but rather a need to survive in a particular environment. Although such a theory would help to explain the drive to deny starvation and continue exercising, it does not entirely explain how exercise becomes so appealing that the person begins to over-exercise in the first place. One putative explanation is offered by reticular-activating hypofrontality (RAH). This neurological mechanism evolved to prevent emotional processing from interrupting the core mechanisms of survival (i.e., motor execution) [21]. This suggests that the experience of emotion is too great a threat to survival, and therefore when a person is exercising, this mechanism is temporarily shut down. Thus it is possible that over-exercise may be a perpetuating, evolution-linked factor for eating disorders.

Alternative theories attach more importance to other realms of the human condition. For instance, the cognitive model suggests that exercise becomes excessive and problematic (i.e., affects the person's quality of life) when it is used as a way to cope with cognitive stress [22]. Once the individual becomes habituated to such a strategy, they then rely on exercise to relieve stress as their main coping strategy. This creates further difficulties in that if the individual is no longer able to exercise, they have few if any effective coping strategies at their disposal. This can have harmful psychological effects, such as experiencing feelings of hopelessness but also being driven to exercise compulsively [23]. Excessive exercise often results in weight loss [24]. Over-exercise leads to a decline in the individual's healthy weight range, resulting in starvation syndrome. As body weight decreases, rigid cognitions, emotional blunting, and dysregulation occur, often leading to social withdrawal and isolation [25], thus perpetuating the cycle in which exercise is used as a coping strategy.

Inevitably, the wider systemic influences of Western cultures that endorse a thin 'ideal' body type have a psychological impact. This body ideal often consists of an athletic, toned, and well-defined physique. The individual may develop ego-syntonic beliefs about appearance and specifically exercise that can lead to self-critical thoughts, with attempts to improve the self through changes in body weight and shape [26]. Excessive exercise appears to affect one's perception of the self, motivating one to continue to strive for perfection (through body image) that never materializes [27,28], thus accounting for the drive to continue to exercise excessively.

Several theories have been suggested to explain why this compulsion continues even when signs and symptoms of physical deterioration have developed. A more robust model is based on endorphins, which are endogenous opioids [29]. Opioids are known for their addictive qualities and euphoric after-effects [30]. However, in the brain they are mainly associated with the reward system, which has been shown to be linked to binge eating [31]. The opioid-receptor system plays a major role in determining how rewarding it is to eat excessively or exercise excessively. Research suggests that there is a craving for and addictive quality to the exercising, induced by the replenishment of opioid receptors, and thus stimulating the reward centre in the brain. The brain craves stimulation and reward, thereby inducing the need to exercise [32]. Arguably, although such rewarding effects may cause and establish the behaviour initally, habit formation may then occur and establish compulsive exercise behaviours, despite the fact that the reward/compensation ratio is changing as the behaviour becomes less rewarding and more chronic [33,34].

Thus if exercise has a psychological component (whether as a coping mechanism or in relation to stress relief), coupled with neurological aspects and even evolutionary contributory factors, compulsive and excessive exercise appears to be a major contributory factor in the onset of an eating disorder [7].

Therefore exercise in people with eating disorders appears to have both compulsive and addictive characteristics, and may share the features of behavioural addictions (e.g., gambling addiction). However, it has not been identified as such or as a distinct disorder in its own right in any of the official classification systems. Importantly, such a distinction may not be appropriate. In behavioural addictions the problematic behaviours cannot be better explained by another recognized disorder. This does not seem to be the case with over-exercise in eating disorders, where the behaviour can very often be traced back and psychologically linked to the eating disorder psychopathology.

7.3 Eating Disorders, Over-Exercise, and Problematic Use of the Internet

There is a general trend towards a more robust exploration of problematic use of the Internet and its relationship with body image [35]. Excessive exercise in the form of media challenges, media prompts, or even government campaigns to tackle other health problems (e.g., the rising prevalence of obesity and metabolic syndrome) has been linked to the consumption of 'thinspiration', 'bonespiration', or 'fitspiration' online content [36,37], appearance anxiety [38], weight loss and fitness tracking applications (Apps), and dieting Apps that prompt activity or weight loss management programmes [39–43]. These issues cut across the diagnostic boundaries of mental disorders characterized by distorted views of one's self and/or one's body, including eating, body dysmorphic disorder, obsessive-compulsive disorder, and other related disorders (e.g., muscle dysmorphia) [44]. More research is required to improve our understanding of how people with a distorted image of their own body interact with the online environment, and to further elucidate the relationship between problematic use of the Internet and body dysmorphic disorder, exercise addiction (EA) [45,46], and the internalization of muscular ideals or 'toxic masculinity' [47]. Those at risk of body dysmorphic disorder who exercise excessively also tend to use image- and performance-enhancing drugs (IPEDs), which include a wide range of untested supplements designed to enhance fitness or weight loss, which regrettably are often used without clinical supervision [45,48,49]. The relationship between IPED use and body image was also the focus of much attention during the COVID-19 pandemic, especially in relation to the impact of lockdown measures and changes in fitness practices across many European countries [50]. There were concerns that, during the pandemic, compulsions in the form of excessive repetitive activity might exacerbate the risk of developing eating disorders. The lockdown measures and other lifestyle changes that occurred were considered to be trigger factors for ritualistic and/or safety behaviour, coupled with the loss of individuals' usual safety routines. Despite this concern about the lockdown periods, a longitudinal study in the UK that involved a psycho-socio-economic assessment of pandemic-related effects on eating disorders [51] found that EA levels did not change from pre- to mid-pandemic for individuals who met the criteria for a probable eating disorder mid-pandemic, nor were they a predictive factor for eating disorders mid-pandemic [52]. In another study from the UK it was reported that the association between obsessive thoughts and eating disorders in an eating disorder cohort with elevated exercise traits (high scores on the Exercise Addiction Inventory, EAI), as well as the association between sensation seeking and eating disorders, were partly mediated by problematic use of the Internet [53]. Thus problematic internet use appears to be a significant domain that may partially explain the relationship between eating disorders, over-exercise, and obsessional thoughts or sensation-seeking impulsive traits. Further research is needed to determine whether it helps to mediate the development and maintenance of excessive exercise as a symptom in eating disorder populations.

7.4 Management of Exercise in Populations with Eating Disorders

It is important that the management and treatment of excessive exercise address the neurobiological and psychological factors involved in the continued use of excessive exercise. One study found that despite recovery from an eating disorder, the psychological impact on the individual was significant, highlighting the importance of measuring and addressing not only the physical state but also the psychological state [54]. Despite physical effects, the cognitive appraisal of the exercise has been found to correlate with the rate of usage. Therefore cognitive approaches have been the first line of treatment when addressing excessive exercise in eating disorder pathology [55].

Guidance from the National Institute for Health and Care Excellence (NICE) recommends that individual cognitive–behavioural therapy (CBT) should be the first-line treatment for individuals with anorexia nervosa, and that a CBT-orientated guided self-help approach should be adopted for bulimia nervosa and binge eating disorder [56]. When a CBT approach is adopted, excessive exercise is often addressed in a gradual manner, with exercise being slowly reduced, cognitive appraisals addressed, and food intake increased. This means that the body will become more nourished and stronger at a pace that is tolerable for the individual. The efficacy of CBT interventions as a treatment for patients with eating disorders is supported by the literature [57–59]. However, a recent systematic review concluded that although body weight increased for individuals with anorexia nervosa, and stabilized for those with bulimia nervosa, driven exercise was not addressed [60]. Furthermore, although outcome measures showed an improvement after the intervention, these results were not sustained, and remission often occurred. Around 50% of those in the bulimia nervosa group were in remission after 5 months. Both groups also showed high attrition rates (20–54%). However, it should be pointed out that this diagnosis has a high remission rate across all studies [61]. Given that exercise seems to have a role in perpetuating eating disorder symptoms, there appears to be a critical need for the development of both psychological and physiotherapy-led approaches to treatment.

7.5 Physiotherapy-Based Psychological Interventions for Eating Disorders

A growing body of research suggests that the incorporation of healthy, supervised, and monitored physical activity could result in reduced anxiety and improved mood, improved body image, and a reduced 'drive for thinness', as well as reduced secretive exercise and exercise drive [62–64]. Historically, inclusion of exercise as part of the treatment for eating disorders was considered detrimental, indeed unsafe, due to the high rates of complex medical risks and the lack of clinical exercise guidelines; therefore the guidelines generally advised total abstinence [65]. However, abstaining from exercise when the psychological determinants of dysfunctional exercising have not been addressed might not lead to the best long-term outcomes [66]. There is now emerging evidence to support the inclusion of the psychosocial aspects of dysfunctional exercise, as well as participation in activities in the community, as part of the journey of recovery from an eating disorder [67–69]. These guidelines support the use of a graded exercise programme, and have shown that effectively challenging and changing beliefs about exercise improves treatment outcomes by influencing the individual's attitudes towards exercise.

Due to the high medical risk and mortality rate associated with eating disorders, the inclusion of exercise interventions as part of eating disorder treatment must be supervised and coordinated by a specialist exercise professional, such as a physiotherapist [69], and prescribed in line with medical, functional, and psychological risk assessment. Exercise prescription must also consider the individual's engagement, including their progress with treatment and restoration of body weight. In addition, a graded approach to the inclusion of exercise allows interventions to be tailored specifically to the individual's health status, risk, short- and long-term exercise goals, exercise preferences, and level of fitness, as well as incorporating psychoeducation about the unhealthy aspects of exercise behaviours.

The type of activity chosen is important [62]. Physical therapy interventions (e.g., aerobic exercise, yoga, basic body awareness) have been found to significantly lower scores for eating pathology and depressive symptoms in patients with anorexia nervosa and bulimia nervosa. In addition, recommendations for longer-term health benefits and developing a healthier approach to exercise suggest that treatment could include flexibility, resistance, and cardiovascular training [67], with appropriate medical precautions.

It is recommended that treatment interventions for dysfunctional exercise also include strategies that challenge the habitual (compulsive), rigid, and rule-driven aspects of exercise behaviour (see Box 7.1). During such activity, individuals with eating disorders might experience a reduced mind–body connection. Therefore enhancing body awareness and the body–mind connection through movement is an important element of treatment, during which the patient relearns their own physical and mental cues relating to physical activity [70].

Finally, treatment of dysfunctional exercise must also address longer-term lifestyle goals and preferences, as well as the opportunity for progression of treatment into community settings, including vocational settings, where the individual can be guided to include appropriate exercise and other physical activity safely as part of a longer-term sustainable and balanced lifestyle. Key factors in achieving longer-term positive outcomes include supporting individuals to include variety, flexibility, and enjoyment as part of a healthy approach to exercise and physical activity [70].

Box 7.1 Summary of aims for management of dysfunctional exercise in eating disorders

Cognitive–behavioural therapy (first-line treatment for anorexia nervosa and bulimia nervosa) incorporates a behavioural graded approach to managing exercise in eating disorders.

A multi-disciplinary approach is adopted, including medical, psychology, and physiotherapy professionals' input, so that the individual's exercise can be formulated within the wider context of their psychosocial difficulties and recovery goals.

The individual's relationship with exercise is described in terms of exercise style, intensity, pattern, and behaviours, and education is provided about healthy vs. unhealthy approaches to exercise.

Psychological interventions are identified and implemented that support the individual to work on their underlying eating disorder psychopathology, with the aim of reducing the need to exercise as a coping strategy.

The individual is supported in challenging their dysfunctional exercise beliefs and rule-driven behaviour, and in engaging with an alternative graded approach to the reintroduction of exercise. Guided exercise that enhances the mind–body connection and signals, and which focuses on social engagement, variety, flexibility, and enjoyment, may be the key to long-term recovery.

The role of problematic use of technology (e.g., social media, fitness/activity tracking devices or Apps) is considered when exploring the factors that maintain dysfunctional exercise in eating disorders.

This chapter concludes by discussing two cases involving over-exercise and disordered eating.

Case 7.1   Janet

Janet is a 28-year-old Caucasian woman with a longstanding history of restricting anorexia nervosa. She has a background of perfectionism and a liking for orderliness in her life, both of which are traits that run in her family. She comes from a high-achieving family who also place value on healthy living, including keeping fit and eating healthy foods. Janet was a star student when she was younger, and has now been working in a law firm for over four years, which has been stressful, and she has often found herself prioritizing work over leisure and self-care. In her early twenties she started to park her car further away from her office so that she could walk to and from work, as many of her friends were talking about how they were trying to walk more in order to get fitter. Janet found that these walks would help her to prepare for the day ahead, or to 'clear her mind' on her way home. Over time she realized how her walking was helping her to manage her anxiety, and she therefore decided to start going for a walk in the evening or at weekends, too. Over the next few years, Janet's walks became longer, more frequent, and faster, and her schedule and routine became more rigid. She found herself working or walking for most of the time, leaving very little opportunity in her life for anything else. She used to enjoy playing the piano, and would attend classical music concerts with a small group of friends. However, she had stopped doing this, as she felt that it would interfere with her ability to meet work targets and would also prevent her from going for her walks. Janet set routines around her walking, and would have to walk the same route at the same time every day. Occasionally she would see one of her friends while she was out walking, but she would not feel able to stop and talk with them due to concerns that she might then not be able to complete her walking route. She was also keen on browsing fitness and walking websites, and she followed a fitness influencer online who promoted the use of step counting. As a result, Janet installed an activity tracker on her phone which included a step counter. She felt that this was a helpful way to keep track of her walking, and therefore began completing a set number of steps each day. She noticed that this gave her a sense of achievement, increased her self-esteem, and helped to reduce the guilt she felt around eating. However, the use of the activity tracker led to further rigidity and routine in her walking. Janet began to feel that she had to earn the right to eat by completing a particular number of steps, and that she would have to reduce her food intake if she had not achieved her daily step goal. She also experienced increasing concern about gaining weight if she was less active, and over time her daily step goals increased.

During an annual health check at work, Janet's occupational health doctor noted that she was losing weight and appeared tired. As a result of their discussion, Janet was referred to the community eating disorder team. She was diagnosed with anorexia nervosa that required further intervention and treatment in the community.

Case 7.1 (cont.)

As part of her treatment, Janet engaged in a physiotherapy assessment to explore her relationship with exercise and the impact that this was having on her physical and mental health. The completion of a scale which measured exercise severity indicated that her exercise was compulsive, and she scored highest in domains that assessed behavioural rigidity and emotional regulation. As part of her treatment, Janet was able to spend time identifying her exercise behaviours and how these were linked to her eating disorder, as well as current maintaining factors for her walking, such as a sense of achievement, permission to eat, feelings of self-worth, and the need to manage stress and anxiety. She admitted that she would like to include activity in her lifestyle, but to do this in a more balanced way. She also mentioned that she had enjoyed walking initially, before it became more driven and rigid, and that she would like to be able to continue walking, but more flexibly and enjoyably.

Janet worked closely with the clinical psychologist to identify alternative ways to manage her anxiety and stress, and to work on the underlying causes of her anorexia so that she could become less dependent on her physical activity as a way of coping. She had used her exercise as a way to manage her anxiety, which suggested that her presentation included cognitive maintaining factors. As this was keeping her burdened with exercising as her main (and perhaps sole) coping strategy, a cognitive–behavioural therapy approach was adopted, which focused on managing emotion and the meaning that Janet gave to her body. The underlying mechanisms that were driving her rigidity were influenced in part by her falling body weight, but also by her family system and values. It would be important to factor in the wider systemic influences on her behaviour in order to empower Janet, rather than to elicit shame and blame with regard to her symptoms.

Alongside this therapy approach, Janet also worked with the physiotherapist to explore her beliefs about exercise and to learn how to identify her anorexia-driven activity and develop a healthy understanding of exercise. She was able to acknowledge that her beliefs about healthy recommendations for exercise had been greatly influenced by her anorexia and perfectionism. She found this work hard, but benefited from a period when she stopped walking and was able to learn the benefits of rest, as well as how to manage the guilt she experienced when not being as active or completing a specific number of steps each day. Janet felt that this allowed her to 'reset', and from that position she was able to experience the enjoyment of movement and exercise through supervised physiotherapy sessions. These focused on body awareness during movement, pace and intensity of movement, and identifying the positive and enjoyable experiences that come from exercise. Janet was able to acknowledge that she had become 'robotic' when walking, over-concentrating on pace and steps, and that she had lost touch with the experience of walking and movement, and what her body was feeling. She was guided to learn how to listen to

Case 7.1 (*cont.*)

her body, both physically and psychologically, and how to understand physical cues such as tiredness and pain so that she could identify when she was not exercising in the right way or at the right time, and make appropriate changes.

At the end of her treatment, Janet joined the walking group in her local community. They met once or twice during the week, depending on their schedules, and once at the weekend. The walking routes and intensity varied, and the sessions were social – they were never about counting steps or monitoring energy expenditure. Janet found that she really enjoyed these sessions and felt that, although they were extremely beneficial for her mental and physical health, she did not need to prioritize them over other social or leisure activities, or take part if she was feeling unwell or tired.

Case 7.2 Brad

Brad is a 23-year-old Caucasian man who attended the accident and emergency (A&E) department to report that he believed he was suffering from bulimia nervosa. He mentioned that he was struggling with his body image, and with low mood, low self-esteem, and loss of confidence. He also disclosed that at times he had considered suicide as a way to end his struggles. During his adolescent years, Brad was very athletic, belonged to many school and college sports teams, and played football and went running with friends at the weekend. He enjoyed his sport and exercise, and gained a great sense of achievement from how well he played, and also self-confidence from being picked for the school and college teams. However, while at school he was also bullied by peers in his year, who called him names for 'wearing poor man's clothes' and not having designer trainers or sports kit, as he was from an impoverished background. After he had finished school, Brad wanted to fulfil his love of sport and dreamed of becoming a football player. He trained regularly, but after sustaining a series of injuries his performance became affected and he felt unable to achieve his dream. Instead, he focused on becoming a personal trainer or a football coach.

Brad also had an Instagram account, and as a result of his posts about his training and sporting achievements he had several thousand followers. The comments of his followers and others online were generally positive, but he did receive some negative comments about his appearance. Brad began to find it difficult to cope with the pressure of being expected to keep fit, or to have an ideal body physique, especially as he experienced periods of feeling emotionally vulnerable and acting on impulse. He declined an invitation to coach at his local football club, as he did not feel he would be good enough. He tried periods of starvation and fasting to burn calories, believing that he needed to

Case 7.2 *(cont.)*

be thinner in order to be fitter and more toned, or to achieve a more athletic build, but he also found that this triggered binge-eating episodes. During his bingeing episodes he would consume more than 10,000 kcal in one meal. These episodes were always followed by self-induced vomiting to get rid of 'the calories' and prevent weight gain. Brad believed that his body image was very important not only for his well-being, but also for his sense of professional achievement and self-esteem. Therefore he decided to use diuretics so as to appear more 'muscular' in the photos that he posted, and he also tried amphet-amines, obtained illegally, to boost his capacity for training. Brad believed that the more he trained, the more toned he would become and the more muscle he could develop. He began to increase his training sessions and push himself to lift heavier weights and complete more sets and reps. He stopped having rest days and would train for longer each day. He stayed late at the gym, long after everyone else had left. The manager of the gym expressed concern about the amount of training Brad was doing, but Brad dismissed this, and moved to a different gym in order to avoid further questioning about his training. A couple of months ago, while training, he sustained a minor tear to the supraspinatus muscle in his shoulder. He went to see a physiotherapist, who advised him to rest and make changes to his training routine while his injury healed. Initially, Brad followed this advice and restricted himself to lower limb weight training exercises. However, he became increasingly concerned about loss of muscle definition in his upper body and about weight gain, so he returned to the gym and resumed his training routine despite the pain and ongoing injury. During a subsequent training session, Brad ruptured his supraspinatus muscle. He was now unable to continue training, so he tried to resume alternative activities such as cycling and running, but found this difficult and felt like a failure. His mood dipped further and he felt unable to cope. His bingeing increased, as did the frequency of purging, and one night he experienced paraesthesia in the form of pins and needles and tingling in his extremities. Brad attended A&E and received intravenous treatment for hypokalaemia; he was also found to have concerning ECG changes related to low potassium levels in his body.

He was admitted to an acute medical ward and received support for priority medical stabilization. He was also referred to the specialist eating disorder unit, and was then transferred there to begin work on the management of his bulimia nervosa. Initially he felt physically weak and unsteady when walking. As both his nutrition and his blood electrolytes improved, his physical strength began to be restored. When he had been feeling weaker, Brad had felt unable to exercise, nor did he feel guilty about resting. However, as he become more medically stable and his strength improved, he began to feel that he should be exercising in order to avoid gaining excess weight or losing muscle mass. He began to exercise secretly in his bedroom, and initially denied this to the team, but he eventually admitted to this behaviour when it was noted that his blood

Case 7.2 *(cont.)*

creatine kinase (CK) levels were significantly raised, indicating that he could be exercising and that muscle breakdown was occurring. Brad became extremely upset, and again felt that he had failed himself. He shared his desperation to recover and not be bound by the rules and beliefs associated with his eating disorder.

As part of his treatment, Brad agreed to take part in a physiotherapy assessment to explore his relationship with exercise and begin exercise management work as part of the therapy approach. Completion of an exercise test showed that Brad's exercise behaviours were compulsive, with the highest score relating to exercise for influencing body weight and shape. The priority for Brad was to ensure that he remained medically stable and to minimize any physical and psychological risks associated with his bedroom exercise. He was able to identify the maintaining factors in his drive for exercise, which included body image and a desire for what he perceived as the ideal physical physique, and the associated sense of achievement and self-esteem. Brad participated in educational sessions about safe and appropriate types, frequency, and intensity of exercise, and the physical and psychological risks of exercise associated with an eating disorder. At the same time, he was given support to enable him to work on his negative body image and low self-esteem.

Individuals with bulimia nervosa are at increased risk of injuries, as many of them engage in dysfunctional exercise. Brad's problematic exercise appeared to be motivated by his belief that the maintenance of his body was very important for his well-being, professional achievement, and self-esteem. Although this belief continued to drive him towards his goal, it also kept him locked in a cycle that left him feeling disappointed, depressed, and hopeless. As well as education about the use of exercise, Brad also received psychoeducation to enable him to understand the vicious cycle of restriction that led to binge-eating episodes, self-induced vomiting, and diuretic use. Due to his underlying beliefs about how his physical appearance determined his well-being and sense of achievement, it was also important for Brad's treatment to include a cognitive–behavioural intervention that targeted these areas. In addition, given his history of others focusing on his appearance and bullying him, it was vital for Brad to create a new narrative focused on who he is and his resilience, rather than on his fragility and need for a sense of achievement.

As part of his treatment, Brad also received support for his ongoing left shoulder injury, and education on how to ensure safe training principles, injury prevention, and recovery. His shoulder injury improved, and after a physical and psychological risk assessment it was considered safe and appropriate for him to begin to take part in supervised and guided low-level gym sessions, with the aim of re-education and exploration of gym-based exercise. However, during this process, Brad realized that he had not enjoyed his previous personal training experience, and that this had been due to the unhelpful coping

Case 7.2 (cont.)

mechanisms that he used to compensate for his lack of self-esteem and his concerns about body image. He was able to identify that it was hard for him to move away from a focus on building physique and gaining acceptance, as he found that the gym environment was an extremely strong trigger of both motives. However, he acknowledged that he enjoyed strengthening exercises as well as cardiovascular exercise, remembering his love of sport and particularly football. Although at this stage Brad's relationship with his body image and self-esteem was improving, exercise management aimed to support him in finding an exercise that he enjoyed, and that moved away from his past exercise goals and experiences. He was allowed to try a series of different exercising opportunities that were available in the community, and he found that he enjoyed group exercise classes such as circuit training and boot camp workouts. He also began to coach at his local youth football club, where he rediscovered his love of football and gained a sense of achievement and enjoyment from coaching others. He also ensured that as part of his coaching he taught healthy exercise principles and how to develop self-confidence through enjoyment of the sport.

References

1   Austin SB. A public health approach to eating disorders prevention: it's time for public health professionals to take a seat at the table. *BMC Public Health* 2012; 12: 854.

2   Erskine HE, Whiteford HA, Pike KM. The global burden of eating disorders. *Curr Opin Psychiatry* 2016; 29: 346–53.

3   Arcelus J, Mitchell AJ, Wales J, Nielsen S. Mortality rates in patients with anorexia nervosa and other eating disorders. A meta-analysis of 36 studies. *Arch Gen Psychiatry* 2011; 68: 724–31.

4   Smink FRE, Van Hoeken D, Hoek HW. Epidemiology of eating disorders: incidence, prevalence and mortality rates. *Curr Psychiatry Rep* 2012; 14: 406–14.

5   Treasure J, Zipfel S, Micali N et al. Anorexia nervosa. *Nat Rev Dis Primers* 2015; 1: 15074.

6   Scharmer C, Gorrell S, Schaumberg K, Anderson D. Compulsive exercise or exercise dependence? Clarifying conceptualizations of exercise in the context of eating disorder pathology. *Psychol Sport Exerc* 2020; 46: 101586.

7   Meyer C, Taranis L, Goodwin H, Haycraft E. Compulsive exercise and eating disorders. *Eur Eat Disord Rev* 2011; 19: 174–89.

8   El Ghoch M, Calugi S, Dalle Grave R. Management of severe rhabdomyolysis and exercise-associated hyponatremia in a female with anorexia nervosa and excessive compulsive exercising. *Case Rep Med* 2016; 2016: 8194160.

9   Peñas-Lledó E, Vaz Leal FJ, Waller G. Excessive exercise in anorexia nervosa and bulimia nervosa: relation to eating characteristics and general psychopathology. *Int J Eat Disord* 2002; 31: 370–5.

10 Delimaris I. Potential adverse biological effects of excessive exercise and overtraining among healthy individuals. *Acta Medica Martiniana* 2014; 14: 5–12.

11 Mitchison D, Mond J. Epidemiology of eating disorders, eating disordered behaviour, and body image disturbance in males: a narrative review. *J Eat Disord* 2015; 3: 1–9.

12 Rizk M, Lalanne C, Berthoz S, Kern L, Godart N. Problematic exercise in anorexia nervosa: testing potential risk factors against different definitions. *PLoS ONE* 2015; 10: e0143352.

13 Strober M, Freeman R, Morrell W. The long-term course of severe anorexia nervosa in adolescents: survival analysis of recovery, relapse, and outcome predictors over 10–15 years in a prospective study. *Int J Eat Disord* 1997; 22: 339–60.

14 Tsai G. Eating disorders in the Far East. *Eat Weight Disord* 2000; 5: 183–97.

15 Miller MN, Pumariega AJ. Culture and eating disorders: a historical and cross-cultural review. *Psychiatry* 2001; 64: 93–110.

16 Holderness C, Brooks-Gunn J, Warren M. Eating disorders and substance use. *Med Sci Sport Exerc* 1994; 26: 297–302.

17 Garner DM, Garfinkel PE. Socio-cultural factors in the development of anorexia nervosa. *Psychol Med* 1980; 10: 647–56.

18 Mond JM, Hay PJ, Rodgers B, Owen C. An update on the definition of "excessive exercise" in eating disorders research. *Int J Eat Disord* 2006; 39: 147–53.

19 Mountjoy M, Sundgot-Borgen J, Burke L et al. The IOC consensus statement: beyond the Female Athlete Triad—Relative Energy Deficiency in Sport (RED-S). *Br J Sports Med* 2014; 48: 491–7.

20 Guisinger S. Adapted to flee famine: adding an evolutionary perspective on anorexia nervosa. *Psychol Rev* 2003; 110: 745–61.

21 Dietrich A, Audiffren M. The reticular-activating hypofrontality (RAH) model of acute exercise. *Neurosci Biobehav Rev* 2011; 35: 1305–25.

22 Egorov AY, Szabo A. The exercise paradox: an interactional model for a clearer conceptualization of exercise addiction. *J Behav Addict* 2013; 2: 199–208.

23 Klump KL, Strober M, Bulik CM et al. Personality characteristics of women before and after recovery from an eating disorder. *Psychol Med* 2004; 34: 1407–18.

24 Adams J, Kirkby RJ. Exercise dependence and overtraining: the physiological and psychological consequences of excessive exercise. *Sports Med Train Rehabil* 2010; 10: 199–222.

25 Fessler DMT. The implications of starvation induced psychological changes for the ethical treatment of hunger strikers. *J Med Ethics* 2003; 29: 243–7.

26 Griffiths S, Mond JM, Murray SB, Touyz S. Positive beliefs about anorexia nervosa and muscle dysmorphia are associated with eating disorder symptomatology. *Aust N Z J Psychiatry* 2015; 49: 812–20.

27 Waller G, Cordery H, Corstorphine E et al. Case formulation. In: *Cognitive Behavioral Therapy for Eating Disorders: A Comprehensive Treatment Guide.* Cambridge University Press, 2013: 96–113.

28 Fairburn CG, Cooper Z, Shafran R. Cognitive behaviour therapy for eating disorders: a "transdiagnostic" theory and treatment. *Behav Res Ther* 2003; 41: 509–28.

29 Leuenberger A. Endorphins, exercise, and addictions: a review of exercise dependence. *Impulse* 2006; 3: 1–9.

30 Riley AL. The paradox of drug taking: the role of the aversive effects of drugs. *Physiol Behav* 2011; 103: 69–78.

31 Giuliano C, Cottone P. The role of the opioid system in binge eating disorder. *CNS Spectr* 2015; 20: 537–45.

32 Weinstein A, Weinstein Y. Exercise addiction - diagnosis, bio-psychological mechanisms and treatment issues. *Curr Pharm Des* 2014; 20: 4062–9.

33 Everitt BJ, Robbins TW. Neural systems of reinforcement for drug addiction: from actions to habits to compulsion. *Nat Neurosci* 2005; 8: 1481–9.

34 Brand M, Wegmann E, Stark R et al. The Interaction of Person-Affect-Cognition-Execution (I-PACE) model for addictive behaviors: update, generalization to addictive behaviors beyond internet-use disorders, and specification of the process character of addictive behaviors. *Neurosci Biobehav Rev* 2019; 104; 1–10.

35 Ioannidis K, Chamberlain SR. Digital hazards for feeding and eating: what we know and what we don't. *Curr Psychiatry Rep* 2021; 23: 1–8.

36 Carrotte ER, Vella AM, Lim MSC. Predictors of "liking" three types of health and fitness-related content on social media: a cross-sectional study. *J Med Internet Res* 2015; 17: e205.

37 Quesnel DA, Cook B, Murray K, Zamudio J. Inspiration or thinspiration: the association among problematic internet use, exercise dependence, and eating disorder risk. *Int J Ment Health Addict* 2018; 16: 1113–24.

38 Corazza O, Simonato P, Demetrovics Z et al. The emergence of Exercise Addiction, Body Dysmorphic Disorder, and other image-related psychopathological correlates in fitness settings: a cross sectional study. *PLoS ONE* 2019; 14: e0213060.

39 Almenara CA, Machackova H, Smahel D. Sociodemographic, attitudinal, and behavioral correlates of using nutrition, weight loss, and fitness websites: an online survey. *J Med Internet Res* 2019; 21: e10189.

40 Embacher Martin K, McGloin R, Atkin D. Body dissatisfaction, neuroticism, and female sex as predictors of calorie-tracking app use amongst college students. *J Am Coll Health* 2018; 66: 608–16.

41 Levinson CA, Fewell L, Brosof LC. My Fitness Pal calorie tracker usage in the eating disorders. *Eat Behav* 2017; 27: 14–16.

42 Linardon J, Messer M. My Fitness Pal usage in men: associations with eating disorder symptoms and psychosocial impairment. *Eat Behav* 2019; 33: 13–17.

43 Simpson CC, Mazzeo SE. Calorie counting and fitness tracking technology: associations with eating disorder symptomatology. *Eat Behav* 2017; 26: 89–92.

44 Ioannidis K, Taylor C, Holt L et al. Problematic usage of the internet and eating disorder and related psychopathology: a multifaceted, systematic review and meta-analysis. *Neurosci Biobehav Rev* 2021; 125: 569–81.

45 Catalani V, Negri A, Townshend H et al. The market of sport supplement in the digital era: a netnographic analysis of perceived risks, side-effects and other safety issues. *Emerg Trends Drugs Addict Health* 2021; 1; 100014.

46 Cataldo I, De Luca I, Giorgetti V et al. Fitspiration on social media: body-image and other psychopathological risks among young adults. A narrative review. *Emerg Trends Drugs Addict Health* 2021; 1; 100010.

47 Rodgers RF, Slater A, Gordon CS et al. A biopsychosocial model of social media use and body image concerns, disordered eating, and muscle-building behaviors among adolescent girls and boys. *J Youth Adolesc* 2020; 49: 399–409.

48 Mooney R, Simonato P, Ruparelia R et al. The use of supplements and performance and image enhancing drugs in fitness settings: an exploratory cross-sectional investigation in the United Kingdom. *Hum Psychopharmacol* 2017; 32: e2619.

49 Corazza O, Roman-Urrestarazu A. *Handbook of Novel Psychoactive Substances: What Clinicians Should Know about NPS.* Routledge, 2019.

50 Dores AR, Carvalho IP, Burkauskas J et al. Exercise and use of enhancement drugs at the time of the COVID-19 pandemic: a multicultural study on coping strategies during self-isolation and related risks. *Front Psychiatry* 2021; 12: 648501.

51 Hampshire A, Hellyer PJ, Soreq E et al. Associations between dimensions of behaviour, personality traits, and mental-health during the COVID-19 pandemic in the United Kingdom. *Nat Commun* 2021; 12: 4111.

52 Ioannidis K, Hook RW, Wiedemann A et al. Associations between COVID-19 pandemic impact, dimensions of behavior and eating disorders: a longitudinal UK-based study. *Compr Psychiatry* 2022; 115: 152304.

53 Ioannidis K, Hook RW, Grant JE et al. Eating disorders with over-exercise: a cross-sectional analysis of the mediational role of problematic usage of the internet in young people. *J Psychiatr Res* 2021; 132: 215–22.

54 Bardone-Cone AM, Higgins MK, St George SM et al. Behavioral and psychological aspects of exercise across stages of eating disorder recovery. *Eat Disord* 2016; 24: 424–39.

55 Bratland-Sanda S, Sundgot-Borgen J, Rø Ø et al. Physical activity and exercise dependence during inpatient treatment of longstanding eating disorders: an exploratory study of excessive and non-excessive exercisers. *Int J Eat Disord* 2010; 43: 266–73.

56 National Institute for Health and Care Excellence. *Eating Disorders: Recognition and Treatment.* NICE guideline [NG69]. National Institute for Health and Care Excellence, 2020. www.nice.org.uk/guidance/ng69

57 Hay P. A systematic review of evidence for psychological treatments in eating disorders: 2005–2012. *Int J Eat Disord* 2013; 46: 462–9.

58 De Jong M, Schoorl M, Hoek HW. Enhanced cognitive behavioural therapy for patients with eating disorders: a systematic review. *Curr Opin Psychiatry* 2018; 31: 436–44.

59 Dalle Grave R, Calugi S, Sartirana M, Sermattei S, Conti M. Enhanced cognitive behaviour therapy for adolescents with eating disorders: a systematic review of current status and future perspectives. *IJEDO* 2021; 3; 1–11.

60 Atwood ME, Friedman A. A systematic review of enhanced cognitive behavioral therapy (CBT-E) for eating disorders. *Int J Eat Disord* 2020; 53: 311–30.

61 Richard M, Bauer S, Kordy H. Relapse in anorexia and bulimia nervosa—a 2.5-year follow-up study. *Eur Eat Disord Rev* 2005; 13: 180–90.

62 Vancampfort D, Vanderlinden J, De Hert M et al. A systematic review of physical therapy interventions for patients with anorexia and bulimia nervosa. *Disabil Rehabil* 2014; 36: 628–34.

63 Ng LWC, Ng DP, Wong WP. Is supervised exercise training safe in patients with anorexia nervosa? A meta-analysis. *Physiotherapy* 2013; 99: 1–11.

64 Quesnel DA, Libben M, Oelke ND et al. Is abstinence really the best option? Exploring the role of exercise in the treatment and management of eating disorders. *Eat Disord* 2018; 26: 290–310.

65 Davis C, Kennedy SH, Ravelski E, Dionne M. The role of physical activity in the development and maintenance of eating disorders. *Psychol Med* 1994; 24: 957–67.

66 Carter JC, Blackmore E, Sutandar-Pinnock K, Woodside DB. Relapse in anorexia nervosa: a survival analysis. *Psychol Med* 2004; 34: 671–9.

67 Cook BJ, Wonderlich SA, Mitchell JE et al. Exercise in eating disorders treatment: systematic review and proposal of guidelines. *Med Sci Sports Exerc* 2016; 48: 1408–14.

68 Scottish Intercollegiate Guidelines Network. *SIGN164: Eating Disorders. A National Clinical Guideline.* NHS Scotland., 2022. www.sign.ac.uk/media/1920/sign-164-eating-disorders.pdf

69 Dobinson A, Cooper M, Quesnel D. *Safe Exercise at Every Stage (SEES) Guideline: A Clinical Tool for Treating and Managing Dysfunctional Exercise in Eating Disorders.* SEES, 2020.

70 Calogero RM, Pedrotty-Stump KN. Incorporating exercise into eating disorder treatment and recovery: cultivating a mindful approach. In: Maine M, Hartman McGilley B, Bunnell D, eds. *Treatment of Eating Disorders: Bridging the Research-Practice Gap.* Academic Press, 2010: 425–41.

Chapter

8

Exercise and the Use of Image- and Performance-Enhancing Drugs within the Gym Environment

Jim McVeigh, Martin Chandler, and Gemma Anne Yarwood

8.1 Context

Drugs to aid performance or change appearance are not a new phenomenon, and there is evidence of various such practices throughout history. In the modern era, the use of drugs to lose weight, to increase muscle size and strength, and to 'revitalize manhood' and increase virility has been well documented [1]. Although concerns were raised in the early twentieth century about the use of such 'secret remedies', no attempt was made to categorize these substances until the early twenty-first century [1].

The term *human enhancement drugs (HEDs)* was coined to define drugs used for a functional purpose rather than for pleasure or gratification due to their psychoactive properties. HEDs have also been described as drugs that support attempts to exceed one's natural potential [2] or to perform 'better than well' [3].

This chapter will focus on drugs that are commonly referred to as *image- and performance- enhancing drugs (IPEDs)* (see Table 8.1), including those taken to enhance musculature, such as anabolic-androgenic steroids (AAS), as well as several associated drugs. It is important to note that many IPED users may use additional HEDs (e.g., to enhance sexual performance, to promote sunless tanning), together with prescription and over-the-counter medications, and also potentially psychoactive drugs.

From the mid-twentieth century, the media and much of society have been far more concerned about the use of IPEDs for doping or cheating within an elite sporting context than with their use being a public health issue within the general population [4]. However, during the last 30 years there have been unprecedented advances in pharmacology, technology, and transportation, together with the development and expansion of the Internet [1]. These advances have directly contributed to IPEDs becoming commonplace within the gym culture worldwide [5]. The scale of the use of these drugs, combined with their potential to cause harm, has become an emerging public health concern [4–7].

Table 8.1 Classification of human enhancement drugs

Drug category	Examples of specific drugs
Musculature[a]	Anabolic steroids, growth hormone
Weight loss[a]	Clenbuterol, 2,4-dinitrophenol (DNP)
Skin and hair appearance[b]	Melanotan II, Latisse, mercury-containing creams
Sexual function[b]	Sildenafil, bremelanotide, yohimbine
Cognitive function[b]	Methylphenidate, modafinil, piracetam
Mood and social behaviour[b]	Fluoxetine, beta-blockers, diazepam

[a] IPEDs used within the gym environment.
[b] Not specific to the gym environment.

8.2 Anabolic-Androgenic Steroids

It is well documented that AAS have become the mainstay of IPED use. Although there is a growing pharmacopoeia of substances that have been used in an attempt to increase muscle size and strength, for over 60 years AAS have remained the first choice of drug [8]. However, the practice of consuming substances in an attempt to achieve muscular enhancement can be found throughout history, and dates back to ancient civilizations such as those of Greece and the Roman Empire [1]. Although the veracity of some accounts may be questioned, they reflect a common drive for muscular enhancement over time and across cultures [9]. The modern era of drug use to enhance muscle size and strength can be traced back to pharmacological advances in the early twentieth century [10]. It was the isolation and synthesis of testosterone in the 1930s that led to the development of AAS in both oral and injectable formulations [11].

All AAS can be defined in terms of their anabolic/androgenic ratio, where the term 'anabolic' refers to the primary muscle-building effect and the term 'androgenic' refers to the secondary effects (e.g., growth of body hair, deepening of the voice, increase in libido). Disassociation of the androgenic component has never been completely achieved [12], but the androgenic properties are of particular concern. In women they have potential masculinizing effects, referred to as virilization [13], and in men the more androgenic anabolic steroids easily become converted to oestrogen (a process called 'aromatization'), resulting in side effects such as gynaecomastia (the development of female breast tissue) [14]. Those AAS that do not aromatize are considered to be much weaker [8]. The half-lives of AAS vary depending on their chemical formulation, ranging from a few hours for some oral AAS (e.g., methandrostenolone) to a week or more for some injectable

Table 8.2 Commonly used anabolic-androgenic steroids (AAS)

Generic name	Common trade name	Usage[a]	Typical dosage (men)[b]
Oral AAS			
Methandrostenolone	Dianabol, Pronabol	56%	15–30 mg/day
Oxandrolone	Anavar	47%	15–25 mg/day
Oxymetholone	Anadrol, Anapolon	36%	50–100 mg/day
Stanozolol	Winstrol	29%	15–25 mg/day
Mesterolone	Proviron	13%	15–150 mg/day
Injectable AAS			
Testosterone enanthate	Delatestryl	55%	200–600 mg/week
Nandrolone	Deca Durabolin	53%	200–600 mg/week
Testosterone propionate	Testoviron	42%	200–400 mg/week
Sustanon	–	40%	250–750 mg/week
Testosterone cypionate	Depo-Testosterone	34%	200–600 mg/week
Trenbolone acetate	Finajet	33%	100–300 mg/week

[a] Based on 684 IPED users [18].
[b] Adapted from *Anabolics* [8].

formulations (e.g., testosterone cypionate) [15]. It is these variations in properties that have led users to employ multiple AAS (known as a 'stack') for a given length of time (a 'cycle'), in order to exploit their different actions, and in the hope that the combination of drugs will also work synergistically. [8]. Typically, multiple oral and injectable AAS (see Table 8.2) are used simultaneously, together with other IPEDs (e.g., growth hormone) and drugs to combat the potential adverse effects (here referred to as ancillary drugs) [16,17]. There is little scientific literature to support these regimes, but there is plenty of 'user-led' or 'underground' information on the Internet. Although often unverified, misleading, and potentially dangerous, some 'user-focused' literature (e.g., [8]) is measured and painstakingly researched.

8.3   Human Growth Hormone and Other Peptide Hormones

In recent years there has been a significant increase in the use of human growth hormone within the gym community. In the 1990s, research in the UK indicated that 3–6% of AAS users had used growth hormone in the previous 6 months [19,20]. Less than 20 years later, 32% of respondents stated that they had used it in the previous year [16,18]. This change has been attributed to an increase in availability and a fall in price (from between £6.58 and £20 per IU in the 1990s to between £1 and £8.33 per IU less than 20 years later) [21].

A range of peptides have become available in the last decade, such as CJC-1295 (a growth hormone-releasing factor) [22], Mechano Growth Factor (a variant of insulin-like growth factor, IGF-1) [23], and growth

Table 8.3 Drugs reported to have been used during the previous year

Generic name	Common trade name	Usage[a]	Typical dosage (men)[b]
Anti-oestrogen drugs			
Tamoxifen citrate	Nolvadex	51%	20–40 mg/day
Clomifene citrate	Clomid	34%	50–100 mg/day
Anastrozole	Arimidex	24%	0.5–1 mg/day
Peptide hormones			
Human growth hormone	Norditropin	30%	1–10 IU/day
CJC-1295		3%	100 mcg three times daily
GHRP2/6		10%	100 mcg three times daily
Insulin	Humalog	10%	Varied (e.g., 5 IU)
IGF-1		7%	40–120 mcg/day
Human chorionic gonadotrophin (hCG)		34%	1,500–4,000 every 5 days
Melanotan II		16%	0.5–1 mg/day
Weight loss			
Dinitrophenol (DNP)		4%	200 mg/day
Clenbuterol	Spiropent	34%	20–12 mcg/day
Ephedrine		30%	50–150 mg/day
Liothyronine (T3)	Cytomel	12%	25–75 mcg/day
Levothyroxine (T4)	Eltroxin	6%	25–150 mcg/day

[a] Based on 684 IPED users [18].
[b] Adapted from *Anabolics* [8].

hormone-releasing peptide (GHRP-6), a growth hormone secretagogue [24] (see Table 8.3). These relatively new peptides are additions to the repertoire of established peptides used in association with AAS, such as insulin [25] and IGF-1 [8,25]. Although Melanotan II is also a peptide hormone it has very different actions, primarily as a skin-tanning agent but also with reported effects on sexual functioning [26]. It was first utilized as a tanning agent by bodybuilders, but its use has now spread to the wider population [27].

8.4 Ancillary Drugs

Ancillary drugs to prevent or mitigate the adverse effects of AAS are well established [28,29]. Prescription medications such as tamoxifen (licensed for the treatment of breast cancer) and to a lesser extent anastrozole and clomiphene are used for their anti-oestrogenic effects to combat AAS-induced gynaecomastia [28]. Human chorionic gonadotrophin (hCG) is commonly injected [18,30] in an attempt to stimulate the production of testosterone by the testes following shutdown as a result of AAS use [31].

Weight loss drugs are used to achieve a hyper-lean muscular appearance within bodybuilding [32]. Some of these drugs act as 'fat burners', such as clenbuterol [33] and the infamous 2,4-dinitrophenol (DNP) [34]. Stimulants such as ephedrine or thyroid-related medications such as levothyroxine (T4) and liothyronine (T3) are also commonly used [8,18], and diuretics are used to counter water retention, which is associated with some AAS [8,18]. It is important to note that drugs used to combat the adverse effects of AAS are also used independently of AAS for their pharmacological effects. This is particularly true of weight loss agents such as DNP [32] and clenbuterol [35].

Furthermore, it is important to note that psychoactive drug use is high among some cohorts of IPED users, with research indicating that the prevalence of cocaine use among some groups of IPED users is many times higher than the level in the general population [16,18,36].

8.5 IPED Use as a Public Health Issue

8.5.1 The Extent of IPED Use

Although there is some evidence to suggest that there has been an increase in the self-directed use of IPEDs in the UK over the last 30 years [4,37,38], there are currently no reliable measures of prevalence. Studies in the 1990s reported a lifetime prevalence of AAS of 9.1% for men and 2.3% for women attending gyms [19]. Further research highlighted the variability in prevalence between different types of gym, namely 50.1% within 'hardcore gyms' compared with 15.1% in 'fitness gyms' [20]. This level of prevalence research has never been replicated in the UK.

The Crime Survey for England & Wales (CSEW) reported a prevalence of AAS lifetime use over the last decade of 1.1% (for the age range 16–59 years), equating to 369,000 (range 311,000–427,000) individuals. Figures for recent (previous year) use are considerably lower, at 62,000 (range 38,000–86,000) [39]. However, as noted by the Advisory Council on the Misuse of Drugs, the CSEW has severe limitations, relying on self-reported behaviour via a survey with limited distribution [40]. Over the last 20 years, studies in the north-west of England have revealed that increasing numbers of those who inject AAS are presenting to needle and syringe programmes [4,40,41]. Further research across the north of England demonstrated that the majority of clients attending many of the needle and syringe programmes were AAS users [42].

In the USA, Pope et al. estimated that 2.9–4 million people had used AAS during their lifetime, with 1 million experiencing AAS dependence [37]. Although prevalence studies are rare, Sagoe et al. have made a significant contribution to our understanding of the situation [38], indicating higher levels of AAS use in the West, the Middle East, and South America, and lower levels of use in Africa and Asia. The prevalence of use of other IPEDs remains unknown.

8.5.2 Characteristics and Subgroups of IPED Users

In recent years there have been significant developments in our understanding of typologies of IPED users [43,44]. Based on qualitative interviews conducted in Denmark, the user's approach to risks and the effectiveness of their drug use were used to develop a typology of the user: the 'expert type', the 'YOLO' (You Only Live Once) type, the 'athlete type', and the 'well-being type'. Similar groupings were found in a more recent cluster analysis of 611 male IPED users in the UK [45]. Despite the heterogeneity of IPED use, much of the extant research focuses on young male users of AAS within the gym environment. The evidence shows that there are as many AAS users over the age of 40 years as there are under the age of 25 years [18], as well as female users, but little is known about this group [13,18,46]. As we gain an improved understanding of the motivations for IPED use and look beyond a superficial rationale for image enhancement, a more complex picture emerges of multiple motivations for use, including appearance, strength, well-being, youthfulness, sexual performance, and sport   [18].

8.6 Adverse Effects of IPEDs

8.6.1 Anabolic-Androgenic Steroids

Much of the data relating to health harms is derived from case reports, case series, and cross-sectional studies that are observational [47]. However, in 2014 the American Endocrine Society summarized the harms associated with AAS for several organs and systems of the body [48]. The extent of the potential impact of AAS on the body is summarized in Table 8.4.

Table 8.4 Adverse effects commonly associated with the use of anabolic-androgenic steroids

Type of effect	Examples
Cardiovascular	Atherosclerosis, hypertension, cardiomyopathy, coagulation
Neuroendocrine	Gynaecomastia, prostatic hypertrophy, hypogonadism, withdrawal
Neuropsychiatric	Depression, aggression, mania
Hepatic	Inflammatory and cholestatic effects, peliosis hepatis, neoplasms (rare)[a]
Musculoskeletal	Tendon rupture, rare/potential epiphyseal closure
Renal	Rhabdomyolysis, glomerulosclerosis, neoplasms (rare)
Immunological	Immunosuppression
Dermatological	Acne, striae

[a] Primarily associated with c17α-alkylated oral products.

Additional adverse neuroendocrine effects experienced by women were identified, such as menstrual irregularities and infertility, with further effects reported elsewhere including clitoral enlargement, deepening of the voice, hair loss, and hirsutism [13,46]; this has often led women to adopt different regimes to their male counterparts [18]. There is growing evidence of the impact of AAS on the brain, with identifiable changes in the structure of the brain reported in long-term, high-dosage AAS users [49–51]. These changes include reduced grey matter volume in multiple sectors of the brain and thinning of the cerebral cortex [50], with a negative impact on working memory, speed of processing, and problem solving [52]. Research has also identified comparable brain characteristics in AAS dependence, similar to findings in other dependencies [51].

8.6.2 Harms Associated with Other IPEDs

Although the majority of the evidence for harms caused by IPED use relates to AAS users, growth hormone is associated with cardiovascular, metabolic, and musculoskeletal effects [21,48]. Evidence of harm among users of other peptide hormones is limited. Although there is clearly potential for insulin administration to have adverse effects [53], as yet there is little evidence available within the context of IPEDs. However, the dangers of DNP as an IPED are well documented, with deaths first reported during its period of licence 100 years ago [54]. More recently, both its impact on the bodybuilding community [55] and its spread to the general population have had fatal consequences [34, 56].

8.6.3 Injecting and the Transmission of Bloodborne Viruses

Data from the UK and Australia indicate levels of viral infection among injecting IPED users that are significantly higher than the levels in the general population [57]. For some populations of injecting IPED users, levels of HIV infection have been found to be comparable to those among opiate injectors [16]. The extent to which these findings can be generalized is not known, nor has it been established whether the transmission is through sexual activity or current/previous injecting [16]. However, these data together with low levels of awareness of hepatitis C infection[58] mean that bloodborne viral infections are a cause for public health concern [59].

8.6.4 The IPED Market

Both the Internet and the gym owner/manager play pivotal roles in the IPED market [60,61], which for some can potentially be highly lucrative [62]. However, much of the market could be described as 'social supply' or 'minimally commercial supply' [60,63], with some suppliers drifting into commercial activity [64]. It is important to note that the internet trade in AAS and other enhancement drugs is just one aspect of a growing global market of illicit sedatives, opioid analgesics, antibiotics, psychiatric drugs, fertility drugs, and stimulants [65], together with an expanding range of novel psychoactive substances [66].

There are long-standing and well-documented public health concerns about the illicit IPED market, which include the accidental or deliberate substitution or addition of active ingredients, gross deviations from the stated dose strength, and contamination with foreign particles or infectious agents [8,47].

Fuelled by low-cost manufacturing in countries such as China and India and by online communication, there has been an exponential rise in the availability of illicitly manufactured drugs [1]. Counterfeit and 'underground-laboratory' products are not restricted to AAS, but include peptide hormones [24,67], ancillary drugs [68], and contaminated supplements [69,70]. This has led to speculation that legitimately produced IPEDs are rarely available [71], and the unknown and unpredictable ingredients of these products are a significant danger to health.

8.7 Responses to the Public Health Issue of IPED Use

8.7.1 Legislation and Controls

There are significant differences in the legal status of AAS and other IPEDs around the world, although most countries have at least some form of restriction on the unlicensed manufacture and supply of IPEDs [1]. In 1996, AAS (together with associated drugs, such as growth hormone and clenbuterol) were placed under the control of the UK Misuse of Drugs Act (1971) as a Class C drug. However, rather than 'criminalising users and further pushing the issue underground' [40], a new subcategory of Class C was created, making it legal to possess AAS for personal use but illegal to engage in unlicensed manufacture or supply of the drug. In subsequent reviews, this status was maintained, although sentences for supply offences were increased and the importation of even small amounts of drugs via the Internet or postal system was prohibited [40].

Across Europe, there are a variety of controls on IPEDs. In countries such as Belgium, it is illegal to possess AAS [72]. In Norway, both use and possession of AAS are illegal [73]. In Cyprus, legislation has been expanded to cover possession of any substances that are on the World Anti-Doping Agency banned list [74]. The USA passed legislation in 1988 classing unlawful supply as a felony. However, prior to this, personal possession of AAS without a prescription was already classed as unlawful in all 50 states [75]. In Australia, steroids are now classed alongside heroin and cocaine in the highest category of dangerous illicit drugs [76].

8.7.2 Prevention and Education

There is little evidence for effective strategies to prevent IPED use [77]. Despite this, National Anti-Doping Organizations (NADOs) are increasingly engaging in doping prevention in recreational sports and in some cases in those individually engaged in exercise [74]. Although doping control strategies (e.g., drug testing in gyms) have been attempted in countries such as Denmark[78], provision of information and education is the more common approach [74], with countries such as Norway employing effective engagement strategies [79]. There are significant challenges facing those who are looking to develop effective interventions to combat the current 'dopogenic' environment [80], with a need to act upon the multiple layers of influence that determine the decision to use IPEDs, from the individual to the societal level [81].

8.7.3 Treatment

The evidence base for effective treatments for IPED users is also limited. Although there are numerous case reports of interventions that have been used to treat the physical and psychological adverse effects of AAS, there is scant evidence relating to the effective cessation of IPED use or to relapse prevention [82]. Some studies have identified multiple barriers to service engagement for IPED users [83], but significant numbers of these individuals may already be engaged in treatment for other substance use issues.

The UK and to some extent Australia have seen increasing numbers of AAS users presenting to needle and syringe programmes, although there is still little evidence as to the most effective methods of delivering these interventions or improving health outcomes for this population [84], despite their overall appetite for health monitoring and support [85].

8.7.4 A Sentinel Population

The numbers of people who are using IPEDs, together with the potential adverse effects of these drugs, makes the development of effective interventions a clear necessity. A prerequisite for any successful intervention is meaningful engagement. Effective interaction will not only facilitate effective engagement with AAS users but also offer wider public health benefits. There are growing numbers of examples of drug use practices (including the use of Melanotan II, DNP and GHB) spreading from AAS users to the general population – to the extent that AAS users, especially the influential bodybuilders, may be considered a sentinel population. Monitoring trends within this population of users may act as an 'early warning system' for drug use in wider society, enabling the early development of health-related strategies [86].

References

1   Evans-Brown M, McVeigh J, Perkins C, Bellis M. *Human Enhancement Drugs: The Emerging Challenges to Public Health.* North West Public Health Observatory, 2012.

2   Van de Ven K, Mulrooney K, McVeigh J. An introduction to human enhancement drugs. In: van de Ven K, Mulrooney K, McVeigh J, eds. *Human Enhancement Drugs.* Routledge, 2020: 1–10.

3   Elliott C. *Better Than Well: American Medicine Meets the American Dream.* W. W. Norton & Company, 2004.

4   McVeigh J, Begley E. Anabolic steroids in the UK: an increasing issue for public health. *Drugs Educ Prev Pol* 2017; 24: 278–85.

5   Sagoe D, Molde H, Andreassen CS, Torsheim T, Pallesen S. The global epidemiology of anabolic-androgenic steroid use: a meta-analysis and meta-regression analysis. *Ann Epidemiol* 2014; 24: 383–98.

6   Kanayama G, Kaufman MJ, Pope HG. Public health impact of androgens. *Curr Opin Endocrinol Diabetes Obes* 2018; 25: 218–23.

7   McVeigh J, Evans-Brown M, Bellis MA. Human enhancement drugs and the pursuit of perfection. *Adicciones* 2012; 24: 185–90.

8   Llewellyn W. *Anabolics*, 11th ed. Molecular Nutrition, 2017.

9   Taylor WN. *Macho Medicine.* McFarland and Company, 1991.

10 De Kruif P. *The Male Hormone.* Brace and Company, 1945.

11 Koch FC. The chemistry and biology of male sex hormones. *Bull N Y Acad Med* 1938; 14: 655–80.

12 Kicman AT. Pharmacology of anabolic steroids. *Br J Pharmacol* 2008; 154: 502–21.

13 Havnes IA, Jorstad ML, Innerdal I, Bjornebekk A. Anabolic-androgenic steroid use among women – a qualitative study on experiences of masculinizing, gonadal and sexual effects. *Int J Drug Policy* 2021; 95: 102876.

14 Friedl KE, Yesalis CE. Self-treatment of gynecomastia in bodybuilders who use anabolic steroids. *Phys Sportsmed* 1989; 17: 67–79.

15 Kicman AT. Pharmacology of anabolic steroids. *Br J Pharmacol* 2008; 154: 502–21.

16 Hope VD, McVeigh J, Marongiu A et al. Prevalence of, and risk factors for, HIV, hepatitis B and C infections among men who inject image and performance enhancing drugs: a cross-sectional study. *BMJ Open* 2013; 3: e003207.

17 Evans-Brown M, McVeigh J. Anabolic steroid use in the general population of the United Kingdom. In: Moller V, McNamee M, Dimeo P, eds. *Elite Sport, Doping and Public Health.* University Press of Southern Denmark, 2010: 75–97.

18 Begley E, McVeigh J, Hope V et al. *Image and Performance Enhancing Drugs 2016 National Survey Results.* Public Health Institute, Liverpool John Moores University, 2017.

19 Korkia P, Stimson GV. *Anabolic Steroid Use in Great Britain: An Exploratory Investigation. Final Report to the Departments of Health for England, Scotland and Wales.* Centre for Research on Drugs and Health Behaviour, 1993.

20 Lenehan P, Bellis MA, McVeigh J. A study of anabolic steroid use in the North West of England. *J Perform Enhanc Drugs* 1996; 1: 57–70.

21 Evans-Brown M, McVeigh J. Injecting human growth hormone as a performance-enhancing drug—perspectives from the United Kingdom. *J Subst Use* 2009; 14: 267–88.

22 Teichman SL, Neale A, Lawrence B et al. Prolonged stimulation of growth hormone (GH) and insulin-like growth factor I secretion by CJC-1295, a long-acting analog of GH-releasing hormone, in healthy adults. *J Clin Endocrinol Metab* 2006; 91: 799–805.

23 Matheny RW Jr, Nindl BC, Adamo ML. Minireview: Mechano-growth factor: a putative product of IGF-I gene expression involved in tissue repair and regeneration. *Endocrinology* 2010; 151: 865–75.

24 Kimergard A, McVeigh J, Knutsson S, Breindahl T, Stensballe A. Online marketing of synthetic peptide hormones: poor manufacturing, user safety, and challenges to public health. *Drug Test Anal* 2014; 6: 396–8.

25 Holt RIG, Sonksen PH. Growth hormone, IGF-I and insulin and their abuse in sport. *Br J Pharmacol* 2008; 154: 542–56.

26 Brennan R, Wells JG, Van Hout MC. An unhealthy glow? A review of melanotan use and associated clinical outcomes. *Perform Enhanc Health* 2014; 3: 78–92.

27 Evans-Brown M, Dawson R, Chandler M, McVeigh J. Use of melanotan I and II in the general population. *BMJ* 2009; 338: b566.

28 Duchaine D. *Underground Steroid Handbook II.* HLR Technical Books, 1989.

29 Phillips WN. *Anabolic Reference Guide.* Mile High Publishing, 1991.

30 Sagoe D, McVeigh J, Bjornebekk A et al. Polypharmacy among anabolic-androgenic steroid users: a descriptive metasynthesis. *Subst Abuse Treat Prev Policy* 2015; 10: 12.

31 Kanayama G, Hudson JI, DeLuca J et al. Prolonged hypogonadism in males following withdrawal from anabolic–androgenic steroids: an under-recognized problem. *Addiction* 2015; 110: 823–31.

32 Ainsworth NP, Vargo EJ, Petroczi A. Being in control? A thematic content analysis of 14 in-depth interviews with 2,4-dinitrophenol users. *Int J Drug Policy* 2018; 52: 106–14.

33 Spiller HA, James KJ, Scholzen S, Borys DJ. A descriptive study of adverse events from clenbuterol misuse and abuse for weight loss and bodybuilding. *Subst Abuse* 2013; 34: 306–12.

34 McVeigh J, Germain J, Van Hout MC. 2,4-Dinitrophenol, the inferno drug: a netnographic study of user experiences in the quest for leanness. *J Subst Use* 2017; 22: 131–8.

35 Milano G, Chiappini S, Mattioli F, Martelli A, Schifano F. β-2 Agonists as misusing drugs? Assessment of both clenbuterol- and salbutamol-related European Medicines Agency Pharmacovigilance Database Reports. *Basic Clin Pharmacol Toxicol* 2018; 123: 182–7.

36 Ip EJ, Yadao MA, Shah BM et al. Polypharmacy, infectious diseases, sexual behavior, and psychophysical health among anabolic steroid-using homosexual and heterosexual gym patrons in San Francisco's Castro District. *Subst Use Misuse* 2017; 52: 959–68.

37 Pope HG Jr, Kanayama G, Athey A et al. The lifetime prevalence of anabolic–androgenic steroid use and dependence in Americans: current best estimates. *Am J Addict* 2014; 23: 371–7.

38 Sagoe D, Pallesen S. Androgen abuse epidemiology. *Curr Opin Endocrinol Diabetes Obes* 2018; 25: 185–94.

39 Home Office. *Drugs Misuse: Findings from the 2018/19 Crime Survey for England and Wales.* Office for National Statistics, 2019. https://assets.publishing.service.gov.uk/government/uploads/system/uploads/attachment_data/file/832533/drug-misuse-2019-hosb2119.pdf

40 Advisory Council on the Misuse of Drugs. *Consideration of the Anabolic Steroids.* Advisory Council on the Misuse of Drugs, 2010. https://assets.publishing.service.gov.uk/government/uploads/system/uploads/attachment_data/file/119132/anabolic-steroids.pdf

41 McVeigh J, Beynon C, Bellis MA. New challenges for agency based syringe exchange schemes: analysis of 11 years of data (1991–2001) in Merseyside and Cheshire, United Kingdom. *Int J Drug Policy* 2003; 14: 399–405.

42 Kimergard A, McVeigh J. Variability and dilemmas in harm reduction for anabolic steroid users in the UK: a multi-area interview study. *Harm Reduct J* 2014; 11: 19.

43 Christiansen AV, Vinther AS, Liokaftos D. Outline of a typology of men's use of anabolic androgenic steroids in fitness and strength training environments. *Drugs Educ Prev Pol* 2016; 24: 295–305.

44 Christiansen AV. *Gym Culture, Identity and Performance-Enhancing Drugs: Tracing a Typology of Steroid Use.* Routledge, 2020.

45 Zahnow R, McVeigh J, Bates G et al. Identifying a typology of men who use anabolic androgenic steroids (AAS). *Int J Drug Policy* 2018; 55: 105–12.

46 Ip EJ, Barnett MJ, Tenerowicz MJ et al. Women and anabolic steroids: an analysis of a dozen users. *Clin J Sport Med* 2010; 20: 475–81.

47 Evans-Brown M, Kimergard A, McVeigh J. Elephant in the room? The methodological implications for public health research of performance-enhancing drugs derived from the illicit market. *Drug Test Anal* 2009; 1: 323–6.

48 Pope HG, Wood RI, Rogol A et al. Adverse health consequences of performance-enhancing drugs: an Endocrine Society scientific statement. *Endocr Rev* 2014; 35: 341–75.

49 Heffernan TM, Battersby L, Bishop P, O'Neill TS. Everyday memory deficits associated with anabolic-androgenic steroid use in regular gymnasium users. *Open Psychiatry J* 2015; 9: 1–6.

50 Bjornebekk A, Walhovd KB, Jorstad ML et al. Structural brain imaging of long-term anabolic-androgenic steroid users and nonusing weightlifters. *Biol Psychiatry* 2017; 82: 294–302.

51 Hauger LE, Westlye LT, Fjell AM, Walhovd KB, Bjornebekk A. Structural brain characteristics of anabolic-androgenic steroid dependence in men. *Addiction* 2019; 114: 1405–15.

52 Bjornebekk A, Westlye LT, Walhovd KB et al. Cognitive performance and structural brain correlates in long-term anabolic-androgenic steroid exposed and nonexposed weightlifters. *Neuropsychology* 2019; 33: 547–59.

53 Ip EJ, Barnett MJ, Tenerowicz MJ, Perry PJ. Weightlifting's risky new trend: a case series of 41 insulin users. *Curr Sports Med Rep* 2012; 11: 176–9.

54 Cutting WC, Mehrtens HG, Tainter ML. Actions and uses of dinitrophenol: promising metabolic applications. *JAMA* 1933; 101: 193–5.

55 Dufayet L, Gorgiard C, Vayssette F et al. Death of an apprentice bodybuilder following 2,4-dinitrophenol and clenbuterol intake. *Int J Legal Med* 2020; 134: 1003–6.

56 Grundlingh J, Dargan PI, El-Zanfaly M, Wood DM. 2,4-Dinitrophenol (DNP): a weight loss agent with significant acute toxicity and risk of death. *J Med Toxicol* 2011; 7: 205–12.

57 Hope V, Iversen J. Infections and risk among people who use image and performance enhancing drugs. In: van de Ven K, Mulrooney K, McVeigh J, eds. *Human Enhancement Drugs*. Routledge, 2020: 85–100.

58 Hope VD, McVeigh J, Smith J et al. Low levels of hepatitis C diagnosis and testing uptake among people who inject image and performance enhancing drugs in England and Wales, 2012–15. *Drug Alcohol Depend* 2017; 179: 83–6.

59 Iversen J, Hope VD, McVeigh J. Access to needle and syringe programs by people who inject image and performance enhancing drugs. *Int J Drug Policy* 2016; 31: 199–200.

60 Coomber R, Salinas M. The supply of Image and Performance Enhancing Drugs (IPED) to local non-elite users in England: resilient traditional and newly emergent methods. In: van de Ven K, Mulrooney K, McVeigh J, eds. *Human Enhancement Drugs*. Routledge, 2020: 230–46.

61 Salinas M, Floodgate W, Ralphs R. Polydrug use and polydrug markets amongst image and performance enhancing drug users: implications for harm reduction interventions and drug policy. *Int J Drug Policy* 2019; 67: 43–51.

62 Forrest A. London man convicted over role in £40m international steroid smuggling gang. *The Independent*, 2019. www.independent.co.uk/news/uk/crime/steroid-smuggling-gang-gurjaipal-dhillon-london-guilty-a8946356.html

63 Coomber R, Moyle L, Belackov V et al. The burgeoning recognition and accommodation of the social supply of drugs in international criminal justice systems: an eleven-nation comparative overview. *Int J Drug Policy* 2018; 58: 93–103.

64 Turnock LA. Inside a steroid 'brewing' and supply operation in South-West England: an 'ethnographic narrative case study'. *Perform Enhanc Health* 2019; 7: 100152.

65 Hall A, Antonopoulos GA. The (online) supply of illicit lifestyle medicines: a criminological study. In: van de Ven K, Mulrooney K, McVeigh J, eds. *Human Enhancement Drugs.* Routledge, 2020: 173–87.

66 Corazza O, Parrott AC, Demetrovics Z. Novel psychoactive substances: shedding new lights on the ever-changing drug scenario and the associated health risks. *Hum Psychopharmacol* 2017; 32: e2616.

67 Stensballe A, McVeigh J, Breindahl T, Kimergard A. Synthetic growth hormone releasers detected in seized drugs: new trends in the use of drugs for performance enhancement. *Addiction* 2015; 110: 368–9.

68 Evans-Brown M, Kimergård A, McVeigh J, Chandler M, Brandt SD. Is the breast cancer drug tamoxifen being sold as a bodybuilding dietary supplement? *BMJ* 2014; 348: g1476.

69 Abbate V, Kicman AT, Evans-Brown M et al. Anabolic steroids detected in bodybuilding dietary supplements – a significant risk to public health. *Drug Test Anal* 2015; 7: 609–18.

70 Thomas A, Kohler M, Mester J et al. Identification of the growth-hormone-releasing peptide-2 (GHRP-2) in a nutritional supplement. *Drug Test Anal* 2010; 2: 144–8.

71 Kimergard A, McVeigh J. Environments, risk and health harms: a qualitative investigation into the illicit use of anabolic steroids among people using harm reduction services in the UK. *BMJ Open* 2014; 4: e005275.

72 Van de Ven K. 'Blurred lines': anti-doping, national policies, and the performance and image enhancing drug (PIED) market in Belgium and The Netherlands. *Perform Enhanc Health* 2016; 4: 94–102.

73 Havnes IA, Jorstad ML, McVeigh J, Van Hout MC, Bjornebekk A. The anabolic androgenic steroid treatment gap: a national study of substance use disorder treatment. *Subst Abuse* 2020; 14: 1178221820904150.

74 European Commission. *Study on Doping Prevention: A Map of Legal, Regulatory and Prevention Practice Provisions in EU 28.* Publications Office of the European Union, 2014. https://ec.europa.eu/assets/eac/sport/news/2014/docs/doping-prevention-report_en.pdf

75 Kleinman CC, Petit CE. Legal aspects of anabolic steroid use and abuse. In: Yesalis CE, ed. *Anabolic Steroids in Sport and Exercise*, 2nd ed. Human Kinetics Publishers, 2000: 333–59.

76 Mulrooney KJD, van de Ven K, McVeigh J, Collins R. Commentary: Steroid madness – has the dark side of anabolic-androgenic steroids (AAS) been overstated? *Perform Enhanc Health* 2019; 6: 98–102.

77 Bates G, Begley E, Tod D et al. A systematic review investigating the behaviour change strategies in interventions to prevent misuse of anabolic steroids. *J Health Psychol* 2019; 24: 1595–612.

78 Christiansen AV. Doping in fitness and strength training environments – politics, motives and masculinities. In: Moller V, McNamee M, Dimeo P, eds. *Elite Sport, Doping and Public Health.* University Press of Southern Denmark, 2010: 99–118.

79 Havnes IA, Jorstad ML, Wisloff C. Anabolic-androgenic steroid users receiving health-related information: health problems, motivations to quit and treatment desires. *Subst Abuse Treat Prev Policy* 2019; 14: 20.

80 Backhouse SH, Griffiths C, McKenna J. Tackling doping in sport: a call to take action on the dopogenic environment. *Br J Sports Med* 2018; 52: 1485–6.

81 Bates G, Tod D, Leavey C, McVeigh J. An evidence-based socioecological framework to understand men's use of anabolic androgenic steroids and inform interventions in this area. *Drugs Educ Prev Pol* 2018; 26: 484–92.

82 Bates G, Van Hout MC, Teck JTW, McVeigh J. Treatments for people who use anabolic androgenic steroids: a scoping review. *Harm Reduct J* 2019; 16: 75.

83 Harvey OA, Keem S, Parriosh M, van Teijlingen E. Support for people who use anabolic androgenic steroids: a systematic scoping review into what they want and what they access. *BMC Public Health* 2019; 19: 1024.

84 National Institute for Health and Care Excellence (NICE). *Needle and Syringe Programmes.* Public health guideline [PH52]. National Institute for Health and Care Excellence, 2014. www.nice.org.uk/guidance/ph52

85 Harvey O, Keen S, Parrish M, van Teijlingen E, Trenoweth S. Support for non-prescribed anabolic androgenic steroids users: a qualitative exploration of their needs. *Drugs Educ Prev Pol* 2019; 27: 377–86.

86 McVeigh J, Salinas M, Ralphs R. A sentinel population: the public health benefits of monitoring enhanced body builders. *Int J Drug Policy*, 2021; 95: 102890.

Bodybuilding, Exercise, and Image- and Performance-Enhancing Drug Use during the COVID-19 Pandemic

Honor D. Townshend and Anna Tippett

9.1 Introduction

The impact of the COVID-19 pandemic was vast and its lasting impact on society will continue to be revealed over the coming years. Both the virus itself and the worldwide government-enforced restrictions that were put in place to curb its spread required significant shifts in most people's daily activities, including health and fitness. Although restrictions varied across the world, the vast majority of countries did not allow access to fitness facilities, with some even enforcing restrictions on the amount of time individuals could spend outdoors exercising. With a significant proportion of the world relying on fitness facilities as their primary exercise space, and not having access to fully equipped home gyms, the shift to a home-based fitness culture drastically altered the nature of and motivations behind fitness.

The overall motivation for these fitness behaviours was shown to have significantly decreased in the first period of lockdown, due predominantly to the lockdown-required changes to behaviours and environments influencing negative situational perception [1]. There is evidence of increasingly innovative methods for achieving fitness, which motivated individuals to maintain their routines [2], and also adaptation of training routines during the first lockdown period by using alternatives, such as lifting heavy buckets and large water bottles in place of gym-based weightlifting [1].

It has also been reported that a significant increase in general consumer engagement with fitness-related content, such as home workouts, live-streamed fitness plans, and even virtual personal trainer sessions has occurred [3]. During this time, both sports organizations and individual athletes had to adapt to using new media technologies to facilitate interactivity. Simultaneously, worldwide preliminary figures show an increased consumption of both traditional and social media formats [3–5]. This, along with the aforementioned adaptation towards home-based fitness culture, meant that how individuals consume and enact individual fitness ideals shifted in subtle but important ways.

The patterns of use of *image- and performance-enhancing drugs (IPEDs)* during this same time period have been found to show similar dramatic changes. The majority of those who report using IPEDs are often involved in bodybuilding and other forms of fitness that require weightlifting, with a key motivator for IPED consumption being to increase strength and develop muscles [6]. However, this also requires the individual to undertake a strength-centric workout routine. Limitations on access to fitness equipment during the COVID-19 lockdowns therefore undoubtedly had an impact on both the physical ability and individual motivation to use fitness supplementation in the form of IPEDs.

In April and May 2020 there were widespread shortages of exported and imported goods worldwide, which also affected illicit markets [2]. *Anabolic-androgenic steroids (AAS)* and the raw materials used in their manufacture were commonly distributed from countries that were hit heavily by the pandemic [2], with a significant proportion of the IPED market involving online purchase from overseas suppliers [7–9]. Another substantial part of the IPED market, namely gyms, also became inaccessible as social sales and distribution [10] were prevented as a result of government-mandated gym closures. As a result it was hypothesized that these major adjustments to the market, as well as limited access to fitness facilities, would lead to difficulty in accessing IPEDs and therefore result in changes to consumption.

9.2 Netnography as a Method for Monitoring Online Platforms

This chapter draws upon a netnographic data collection method, which involves the ethnographic monitoring of online platforms by regular observation [11]. Data were collected from a selection of conversation-based threads across four open-access fitness forums for a period of 6 months in 2020. A total of 115 forum threads were observed, and the data were then subjected to manual thematic and narrative content analyses. This chapter's discussion includes data collected in relation to three of the five themes explored by the studies, namely 'motivation for use (of IPEDs)', 'body goals', and 'general attitudes towards IPEDs use'. All of the forums observed were open access, and any citations utilized are drawn from threads available for public viewing. However, where possible the data have been anonymized to ensure appropriate limits to data use, with quotations being cited either without names or with pseudonyms attached.

Ethical approval for the study was granted by the University of Hertfordshire.

9.3   Fitness Activities during the COVID-19 Pandemic

The following section discusses the impact of the COVID-19 pandemic on fitness generally, as observed in the assessed forums, focusing on physical limitations, routine adjustment, and fitness innovation. Although the physical impact of these behaviours was clearly affected by the pandemic in the immediate lockdowns, the findings discussed here may also be indicative of the development of future longer-term behavioural changes, including the excessive engagement in exercise already observed to date [12].

9.3.1   Physical Limitations

The lack of access to adequate spaces, specialized facilities, and equipment led most regular gym attendees to adapt their workout routines. Research has shown that the nature of lockdowns could foster 'sedentary behaviour', increasing risks not only to physical health but also to mental health [13–15]. Concern about this was reflected throughout the assessed posts across all forums.

Of particular prevalence in this discussion thread was frustration regarding lack of access to equipment for heavy lifting – an activity often associated with bodybuilding and muscle gain – with one forum user stating that 'home workouts, good as they are, can't make up for the heavy lifting that I need to do'.

The physical limitations to fitness were mainly discussed in relation to the posters' concerns about body image maintenance, with one forum user stating 'I've been reduced to the muscle structure of a prepubescent boy'. However, several forum users were also concerned by the potential negative impact on their strength, with one post stating 'I could bench 95 kg pre lockdown BB curl 35 and skull crush 30 but with this lockdown it's going to be different when gyms reopen', and another stating, in opposition to the regulations, 'Keep vulnerable people away from gyms, keep strong people strong'.

However, those concerned about this loss of muscle were critiqued within the forums, with one post stating that 'Obsessively wanting to cling on to muscle mass in the current climate when it can easily be regained at a later date does not sound like the rational option to me and might indicate that you have deeper psychological issues'.

Previous research has highlighted the role of gaining and maintaining strength as a key factor in the motivation for fitness among many men [16], so the frustrations identified in this context support those earlier findings.

9.3.2   Routine Adjustment and Fitness Innovation

Because of the lack of access and reduced levels of fitness motivation [1], many individual fitness routines changed significantly during the pandemic, and these adjustments were discussed extensively in the observed forums. The level of adjustment varied depending on individual circumstances, with some forum posters specifically linking financial affluence to the ability to maintain muscularity and strength during this time. Often, though, the changes included concentrating on more cardiocentric routines and sport-specific activity, as opposed to the reported previous standard among the forum's weightlifting cohort. Attitudes towards such adjustments among forum users varied, and frequently these attitudes appeared to be directly linked with the self-perceived impact on individual posters' body image goals. Some forum users maintained positive attitudes and actively welcomed the change to their routines, with one comment stating that 'a change is good sometimes to keep things fresh and progressing'. In contrast, however, others displayed disappointment, with one comment stating 'I don't have access to a gym, only a few dumbbells, so I won't be able to work at the intensity I'd like'. This suggests that the impact of fitness routine adjustment necessitated by the pandemic varied and was largely dependent on individual circumstances.

It was because of the previously mentioned frustrations and fears about strength and muscle loss that innovative methods for fitness maintenance were developed by many. A study from Germany showed that a diverse range of fitness activities were displayed in response to the physical restrictions imposed by lockdowns [15]. Although a large proportion of individuals (31.1%) scaled down their physical activities or stopped exercising altogether during this period, nearly as large a number maintained their usual levels of exercise (27%), and a third group actively increased their physical activities (5.7%) [15]. With such a substantial number of individuals appearing to at least maintain, if not increase, their fitness levels, and with only a minority of individuals having access to home gyms, it is understandable why adaptation and innovation of fitness activities occurred.

In the assessed forums, one commonly observed response to the imposed physical limitations and the unaffordability of home-gym equipment was the construction of DIY fitness equipment, which included sawing wood, carrying heavy stones, and crafting homemade weightlifting benches. These comments are in line with the hypothesis presented by Barnaby Zoob Carter, Ian Boardley, and Katinka van de Ven, who considered that 'many individuals were able to come to terms with the restrictions and adapt their training regimes and/or training goals to lessen the perceived impact of the pandemic on their training' [2, p. 305]. Such findings evidence both the importance of maintaining fitness routines for regular strength trainers, and the perceived adaptability of these individuals, even during periods of significant societal change.

9.4 Use of Image- and Performance-Enhancing Drugs during the COVID-19 Pandemic

Similarly to how COVID-19 restrictions globally affected fitness generally, the pandemic also had an impact on the use of IPEDs. Both the availability of and access to products, as well as motivation to utilize them, were affected significantly and this was discussed extensively on the observed forums. Several studies have suggested that the significant impact of the pandemic on lifestyle for most of the population may have led to heightened compulsive engagement with exercise practices, and so resulted in increased use of IPEDs [12,17,18]. However, as mentioned previously, there was an observed negative impact on fitness motivation generally, which would suggest that utilization of IPEDs may have decreased. A third possibility combines these two theories – that is, use of IPEDs generally decreases, but among those who do continue to use these substances and maintain (or increase) their fitness levels, there is an increased level of problematic engagement with the chosen substance.

A total of 40 individual comments across 15 separate discussion threads in the observed forums referenced individuals adjusting their use of IPEDs due to the COVID-19 pandemic. Many comments described forum users' frustrations with these necessitated changes, with one forum user stating 'I had to cut short my 12-week cycle by 5 weeks due to this shitty flu virus. Be months before gyms and bars reopen'.

However, in contrast, some users expressed their relief about these necessitated changes, which presented them with an opportunity to reduce or stop their IPED use. One forum user commented 'It's a relief as it finally gives me a reason to come off-cycle'. Another forum user also reflected on the merits of stopping IPEDs use: 'This lockdown has really highlighted the amount of time and money I've pissed away chasing muscle gain and size, etc'. Furthermore, many users communicated their desire to restart interrupted cycles when restrictions were lifted, with one comment stating that the user was 'Definitely going back on cycle once the lockdown is lifted'. These differing opinions suggest that the effects on IPED use over lockdown were not linear, and that more extensive research is required to fully quantify and understand these impacts, both at the time and in the long term.

Many of these cycle adjustments were referred to as side effects of the changes to fitness and workout routines mentioned earlier. However, another element considered was the physical accessibility of the actual products. One comment stated 'My guy can't get gear ATM', with posters then alerting other forum users to the perceived prevalence of fake advertisements. This led to an increase in perceived unreliability of online purchasing of IPEDs, which was arguably one of the only routes of purchase available during the initial COVID-19 restrictions. These unprecedented changes to the market led some forum users to report stockpiling of IPEDs, while others reported concerns about the potential increase in the home-brewing of IPEDs – a practice associated with significant health risks [19]. However, such home-brewing met with significant disapproval on the observed forums, with one comment stating disparagingly: 'Another gammon intent on preparing injectables in his house'.

Although such comments do not provide any indication of the statistical prevalence of these practices, if further research is shown to highlight a significant increase in home-brewing, the risk to public health and changes to supply lines could be significant.

Whereas access to IPEDs and the feasibility of their use went through periods of extensive change due to the COVID-19 pandemic, the reported rationales for use of IPEDs remained constant. Throughout the forums, posters referenced body image, strength, libido, athletic performance, anti-ageing, general fitness, sleep, recovery from injury, improving mental health, and attracting women – none of which are new, with many being identified by Emma Begley, Jim McVeigh, and Vivian Hope years previously [6]. Therefore, despite the significant impact on more practical factors related to IPED use, the observed forums appear to indicate a limited change in reasons for uptake and/or continued use of these drugs.

9.5 Misinformation

One significant area of concern observed in the research was the circulation of misinformation, which has potentially serious implications for public health. Some forum users believed that intake of AAS could reduce the risks of serious health reactions to COVID-19, with one comment stating: 'Low testosterone in males is also being linked to more serious cases. Wouldn't fancy doing a PCT right now!'.

This view was often countered within the threads, with other forum posters suggesting that the consumption of AAS would in fact increase the health risks associated with COVID-19. One example of this was the following comment: 'if someone using gear were to contract the new Corona Virus, they are more likely to become seriously [ill] than if they weren't on' *[sic]*.

This area poses potentially significant health risks due to the unsupported and contradictory claims being made throughout, particularly when there was evidence of some forum users acting on these claims by actively increasing and/or restarting their IPED cycles.

9.6 Conclusion

The inevitable impact of COVID-19 and the associated restrictions on fitness facilities and IPED use is increasingly being demonstrated by research studies generally and by the data observed on the forums for the study described in this chapter. What remains unclear from this research, though, is whether any particular attitude towards the lockdown-necessitated changes in lifestyle and fitness predominated. Significant variations in attitude towards the changes, as well as in methods of adjustment, were observed throughout the forums. Some comments indicated that new and innovative approaches to fitness were being developed, whereas others merely stated concerns and frustration about the impact.

Although it is not yet possible to foresee the longevity of the effects of this time period on both fitness generally and IPED use specifically, the research presented suggests that there were significant changes in self-rationalization, and so may indicate a long-term influence on associated behaviours.

References

1   Kaur H, Singh T, Arya YK, Mittal S. Physical fitness and exercise during the COVID-19 pandemic: a qualitative enquiry. *Front Psychol* 2020; 11: 29–43.

2   Zoob Carter BN, Boardley ID, Van de Ven K. The impact of the COVID-19 pandemic on male strength athletes who use non-prescribed anabolic-androgenic steroids. *Front Psychiatry* 2021; 12: 636706.

3   Hayes M. Social media and inspiring physical activity during COVID-19 and beyond. *Manag Sport Leis* 2022; 27: 14–21.

4   Chao M, Chen X, Liu T, Yang H, Hall BJ. Psychological distress and state boredom during the COVID-19 outbreak in China: the role of meaning in life and media use. *Eur J Psychotraumatol* 2020; 11: 1769379.

5   Goel A, Gupta L. Social media in the times of COVID-19. *J Clin Rheumatol* 2020; 26: 220–23.

6   Begley E, McVeigh J, Hope V. *Image and Performance Enhancing Drugs: 2016 National Survey Results*. Public Health Institute, Liverpool John Moores University, 2017. Available at: www.ipedinfo.co.uk/resources/downloads/2016% 20National%20IPED%20Info%20Survey%20report%20FINAL.pdf

7   Cordaro FG, Lombardo S, Cosentino M. Selling androgenic anabolic steroids by the pound: identification and analysis of popular websites on the Internet. *Scand J Med Sci Sports* 2011; 21: e247–59.

8   Hall A, Antonopoulos G. License to pill: illegal entrepreneurs' tactics in the online trade of medicines. In: *The Relativity of Wrongdoing: Corruption, Organised Crime, Fraud and Money Laundering in Perspective*. Wolf Legal Publishers, 2015: 229–52.

9   van de Ven K, Koenraadt R. Exploring the relationship between online buyers and sellers of image and performance enhancing drugs (IPEDs): quality issues, trust and self-regulation. *Int J Drug Policy* 2017; 50: 48–55.

10 Coomber R, Salinas M. The supply of Image and Performance Enhancing Drugs (IPED) to local non-elite users in England: resilient traditional and newly emergent methods. In: van de Ven K, Mulrooney KJD, McVeigh J, eds. *Human Enhancement Drugs*. Routledge, 2019: 230–46.

11 Kozinets RV. *Netnography: Redefined*, 2nd ed. Sage, 2015.

12 Dores AR, Carvalho IP, Burkauskas J et al. Exercise and use of enhancement drugs at the time of the COVID-19 pandemic: a multicultural study on coping strategies during self-isolation and related risks. *Front Psychiatry* 2021; 12: 648501.

13 Brooks SK, Webster RK, Smith LE et al. The psychological impact of quarantine and how to reduce it: rapid review of the evidence. *Lancet* 2020; 395: 912–20.

14 Lippi G, Henry BM, Sanchis-Gomar F. Physical inactivity and cardiovascular disease at the time of coronavirus disease 2019 (COVID-19). *Eur J Prev Cardiol* 2020; 27: 906–8.

15 Mutz M, Gerke M. Sport and exercise in times of self-quarantine: how Germans changed their behaviour at the beginning of the Covid-19 pandemic. *Int Rev Sociol Sport* 2021; 56: 305–16.

16 Sell A, Hone LS, Pound N. The importance of physical strength to human males. *Hum Nat* 2012; 23: 30–44.

17 Hausenblas HA, Schreiber K, Smoliga JM. Addiction to exercise. *BMJ* 2017; 357: j1745.

18 Wang M, Baker JS, Quan W, Shen S, Fekete G, Gu Y. A preventive role of exercise across the coronavirus 2 (SARS-CoV-2) pandemic. *Front Physiol* 2020: 11: 572718.

19 Brennan R, Wells JS, Van Hout MC. "Raw juicing" – an online study of the home manufacture of anabolic androgenic steroids (AAS) for injection in contemporary performance and image enhancement (PIED) culture. *Perform Enhanc Health* 2018; 6: 21–7.

How to Treat Exercise Addiction

Psychological Interventions and New
Pharmacological Perspectives

Ilaria De Luca, Attilio Negri,
and Giuseppe Bersani

Case 10.1 Peter

Peter is a 37-year-old man who is living with his parents. He has no brothers or sisters. His family is of relatively high socio-economic status, and he experienced no significant traumatic or interpersonal problems during his childhood. He performed well at school, and after obtaining a degree in motor sciences he worked as a PE teacher in a secondary school. His intimate relationships have all been short term in nature, the last one having ended after 2 years. He showed normal adjustment in relation to work and social relationships. His personality traits included intense mood instability and impulse dyscontrol, with a history of previous aggressive behaviours. There was a period of sporadic use of psychostimulant drugs, mainly amphetamines, between the ages of 21 and 29 years, which ended after a major episode of aggression that had judicial consequences.

From the age of 20 years, Peter became increasingly preoccupied with physical fitness, increasing the amount of time he spent in gyms and sports centres, and engaging in challenging physical exercise. After an initial period in which he was monitored by personal trainers, he then for several years made his own decisions as to the type and duration of training that he practised. Over the last 4 years, the time he spent exercising increased until it occupied a large part of the day, with negative effects on his other social activities and interests. His performance at work remained good, but was strictly limited to helping students who were in physical training. During the same period, he reported increasing use of anabolic-androgenic steroids (AAS) and nutritional supplements, without medical prescription or supervision. Consumption of higher dosages of AAS was linked to states of marked irritability, mood reactivity, and insomnia, with increasing problems in his family and social relationships. In the last year, all activities other than work and training were put on hold, and Peter spent the majority of his time in training. Every attempt by his parents, relatives, or friends to alert him to the excessiveness of his behaviour met with very irritated responses, and he stated that physical training and body shaping

Case 10.1 (*cont.*)

were 'the most important objectives of his life'. This goal certainly appeared to be of the utmost importance, as he ceased almost all social contact with his friends or with women. He sometimes seemed to recognize that he was now unable to reduce his training activities, which he experienced partly as compulsive, but mainly as a source of pleasure, but he had no intention of changing his behaviour. At the age of 23 years, Peter started a psychotherapeutic treatment, but abandoned it after a couple of months. Since then, no other psychological or medical assistance had been sought, despite his parents' advice, and he had received no psychopharmacological treatment.

After an episode of extreme physical weakness followed by an aggressive reaction towards his mother, he agreed to be visited by a psychiatrist, to whom he reported his behavioural history and his psychological attitude to physical exercise. At this point Peter recognized for the first time that the condition he was experiencing was a real addiction, and that he was unable to reduce even the most extreme aspects of his behaviour. He refused a new psychotherapeutic treatment that was offered, but then accepted a pharmacological treatment which was aimed at reducing the compulsion to train, improving his mood, and reducing his emotional reactivity. After 3 months of treatment with the antidepressant/anti-obsessive agent fluvoxamine (250 mg/day) and the mood stabilizer/anti-aggression agent valproate (1,500 mg/day), together with low doses of the anti-anxiety agent clonazepam to support sleep, there was a clear reduction in the amount of time Peter was spending in physical training, even though his aim was still to reach and maintain a 'perfect' body shape. There continued to be a compulsive element to his training, but he was much better able to control his compulsions and to alternate times of training with times of rest or involvement in other activities. His mood was improved and more stable, and no episodes of intense reactivity or aggression had occurred.

In the following months, the clinical response was consolidated, despite some short periods in which there was a partial return to the compulsive training, mainly when he was experiencing environmental stress due to family problems. In terms of general outcome, Peter showed a positive response to the treatment, even if the compulsive personality traits remained only partially controlled and continued to influence his lifestyle and behaviour. At this stage he agreed to take part in cognitive–behavioural therapy, as he was aware of the need to explore in depth his psychological style and reactions.

Case 10.2 Tom

Tom is a 28-year-old man who is living with his mother. His parents are divorced. He is in a long-term relationship with a woman, with no definite intention to marry or live together. He works as an engineer, and has high

Case 10.2 (cont.)

socioeconomic status. He is employed by an international company, is very ambitious about his professional career, and very conscientious in his performance at work. Since adolescence he has been much more involved in practical than intellectual pursuits. There are some anxiety traits in his mode of reaction to stress, and he has a history of several short episodes of hypochondriacal responses to mild physical problems. He is always very concerned about his physical appearance, which he admits is associated with an ideal of perfection, paralleling the general expectations regarding his professional and personal development. Narcissistic traits were evident in his personality, but with a substantial positive influence on his behaviour and relationships.

After the age of 26 years, Tom's concerns about his physical health and bodily appearance increased, and he took up running. He increasingly dedicated himself to this activity until he was running during all his free time outside work. This had a negative impact on his personal relationships, including that with his girlfriend. Paying careful attention to his body shape, body weight, and general state of health became his main interest, and he saw no psychological conflict in this, asserting that 'a perfect body and perfect health are the most important factors at the base of a successful life'. He spent increasing numbers of hours after work and most of his days off running in the fields or around the lake near his home. He never asked for any psychological help to address this excessive behaviour, as in his view it was not pathological. His mood was stable and positive, and he did not report any issues affecting the balance of his life.

About 6 months before he finally agreed to a psychiatric consultation, at a time when he urgently needed to make decisions about his future family life, Tom began to complain of muscle pain in his legs, associated with some difficulties with leg movement. This was probably due to overuse, but fearing that it was an early symptom of a progressive neurological disease he underwent many medical consultations and examinations, none of which identified any underlying problems. Finally, under pressure from his parents, he consulted a psychiatrist. At that visit he showed a marked hypochondriacal concern about the muscle problems, which he refused to accept could have been caused by excessive training. He also exhibited narcissistic traits, which appeared quite dominant in his personality profile and strongly influenced both his behaviour and his judgement. Regarding his overtraining and the huge amount of time that he spent running, he stated that this was necessary for his body shape and health as well as for his psychological well-being. He also commented that at present he felt unable to limit the duration of the training, and sometimes forced himself to continue by remembering that any reduction could jeopardize the 'perfect' body shape that he wanted to maintain.

In view of the somatic disturbance that Tom was exhibiting, he was offered and he accepted treatment with low doses of the antidepressant paroxetine to counteract his anxiety and hypochondriacal concern, together with valproate to

Case 10.2 *(cont.)*

reduce the urge to run, and the benzodiazepine alprazolam to promote general relaxation. The symptom response was rapid and positive, resulting in lower levels of hypochondriacal concern and a general calmness, which in turn led to an objective reduction in the amount of time he spent running, although he remained convinced of its fundamental importance. There was a progressive improvement in the muscle symptoms, with complete remission after 4 months of treatment. At this point, Tom agreed to undergo psychological treatment, which aimed to explore the possible mechanisms underlying both his need for perfection and his somatic response to stress.

10.1 Introduction

There is consensus among clinicians that regular physical activity plays a central role in maintaining health and preventing disease [1], a view that has been reinforced by modern social culture and highlighted by the media. Although the physical and psychological benefits of exercise are widely recognized, there is growing evidence that when exercise becomes excessive or uncontrolled it may develop into addictive behaviour, which may pose significant threats to both physical and mental health [2–5]. Reports of 'compulsive exercise' or 'exercise dependence' have appeared in the literature since the 1970s [6,7], describing a phenomenon that has been defined as a 'multidimensional, maladaptive pattern of exercise, leading to clinically significant impairment, or distress' [8]. Subsequently, several diagnostic criteria for exercise addiction (EA) have been proposed [9], although such a condition is not listed in either the tenth edition of the *International Statistical Classification of Diseases (ICD-10)* or the fifth edition of the *Diagnostic and Statistical Manual of Mental Disorders (DSM-5)*. Hausenblas et al. and Downs et al. classified EA mainly on the basis of the criteria for substance dependence listed in the text revision of the fourth edition of *Diagnostic and Statistical Manual of Mental Disorders (DSM-IV-TR)*, namely tolerance, withdrawal, lack of control, intention effects, time spent engaging in the behaviour, reduction in other activities, and continuance of the behaviour despite the emergence of physical, psychological, and/or interpersonal problems [10,11].

In view of its benefits in maintaining or improving both physical and mental health, including the treatment of certain addictions (e.g., smoking, alcoholism, amphetamine misuse) [12–14], it might appear paradoxical that exercise itself can also develop into a serious dependence. The phenomenon has found fertile ground in a society where the habit of exercising – even when excessive or out of control – is usually accepted, unlike most other addictive behaviours, which are commonly stigmatized. Since the 1980s, fitness centres and gyms have facilitated the development of an 'exercise culture' by promoting a sense of belonging to a group and having a social identity, thus helping to make physical activity both a personal matter and a social one [15]. In addition to this, the fitspiration trend promoted by social networks, with constant posting of images of fashionable and 'perfect' bodies, has generated new behavioural trends with both positive and negative implications for health and well-being [16–18] in terms of body satisfaction, exercise behaviour, and mental health. For instance, in 2016 a systematic review reported that the use of any social network is related to body image concerns and disordered eating [19]. Another study, involving a sample of women who regularly posted fitspiration images, showed that they scored higher than the control group on drive for thinness and EA [20]. Such a sociocultural context for EA may lead to fewer conflicts and interpersonal problems with relatives and friends than would be the case for other substance-related or behavioural addictions. It has been suggested that conflict, defined as 'ill feeling and disputes with people immediately around the addict about the harm the excessive activity may be doing to the addict and all concerned', is one of the main diagnostic indicators of behavioural addictions [21]. Andreassen et al. differentiated between productive and unproductive behavioural addiction on the basis of social acceptability [22]. Exercising for many hours a day is considered 'normal', in contrast to 'abnormal' activities such as internet or video-game abuse, compulsive shopping, or gambling [23]. As exercising is considered to be a sign of a healthy and trendy lifestyle, EA tends to be a socially accepted behaviour [24], which may lead to an underestimation of the phenomenon, and frequent underreporting. People who engage in excessive and uncontrolled exercise are more likely to develop overuse injuries (e.g., stress fractures, tendinopathies) [25,26] and symptoms of endocrine or metabolic dysfunction (e.g., anaemia, amenorrhoea, persistent fatigue, sleep disturbance) [27–29]. They may abandon their social, occupational, and family obligations, resulting in both physical and psychological distress [30], or they may report withdrawal symptoms linked to inability to exercise (e.g., restlessness, anxiety, sadness, irritability, inability to sleep, poor concentratration) [31,32]. Furthermore, the constant drive to perfect their body may lead them to use chemical supplements to achieve their objective. The use of AAS and other hormones among athletes and bodybuilders has been well documented since the 1980s [33], but recent studies have reported the availability of a range of new fitness-enhancing substances. Such image- and performance-enhancing drugs (IPEDs) may include proteins, vitamins, natural products, medical products (e.g., diuretics, hormones), and illicit drugs (e.g., amphetamine-like appetite suppressants) [34]. These compounds are often marketed online as safe and natural products, and are consumed by users despite their potential contaminants and associated health risks [34–36]. Furthermore, it has been suggested that EA may co-occur with other addictions, both behavioural (e.g., sex, work, shopping, and Internet addictions) and substance related (e.g., nicotine, alcohol, and illicit drug addictions) [37,38].

EA has high comorbidity and is significantly correlated with eating disorders and body image disorders [39,40]. It has been estimated that more than 40% of people who have eating disorders are also affected by EA [41]. This relationship has important implications for the diagnosis and treatment of EA. In 1995, Veale distinguished between primary EA, defined as a 'preoccupation with exercise that is not better accounted for another mental disorder', and secondary EA, which is manifested in the presence of anorexia and/or bulimia nervosa [42].

Such a complex and dynamic scenario indicates that a better understanding of the phenomenon is needed by healthcare professionals, as the literature on the subject is limited and research is still ongoing, especially with regard to treatment options.

10.2 Psychological and Pharmacological Treatments

This chapter will only consider primary EA, as overtraining in secondary EA is mainly a consequence of anorexia or bulimia, and therefore the main treatment target is the eating disorder itself.

The literature on the treatment of EA is sparse, and there have been no recent studies of the subject. The challenge in treating this addiction lies in the fact that it is impossible to abstain from the habit completely, because physical activity plays a central role in improving and maintaining health. The main goal of therapeutic options for EA is not to prevent the patient from working out, but to help them to recognize their addictive behaviour and reduce harmful exercise patterns [30]. Furthermore, clinicians should pay particular attention to the assessment and treatment of potentially associated conditions (e.g., dysrhythmias, injuries, myocardial fibrosis), as well as to possible comorbid addiction, both behavioural and substance related. In this scenario, a referral to a multidisciplinary team of professionals, including psychiatrists, psychologists, orthopaedic surgeons, endocrinologists, dietitians, and social workers, may be needed.

10.3 Social and Psychological Interventions

10.3.1 Awareness and Education

Awareness and education are fundamental to the management of EA. A study conducted by Adams and Kirkby revealed that practitioners faced a significant challenge in recognizing this condition, mainly because they were not aware of EA and its diagnostic criteria [43]. An inability to identify the problem and provide an appropriate treatment substantially decreases the likelihood of success [44]. Exercise addicts are generally perceived as having a strong sense of dedication and willpower, which may only increase their commitment to working out [45]. Berczik et al. have emphasized the importance of teaching the concepts of self-control and moderation, stating that ideally 'these lessons should be provided by teachers and parents as a proactive measure, but someone addicted to exercise might only learn these valuable facts for the very first time from a physician' [46]. Patients should receive information about the harmful effects of extreme exercise, and should be encouraged to train in a way that allows them to maintain physical, psychological, and social well-being [47]. The recommendations produced by the Canadian Society for Exercise Physiology in 2016 state that 'all apparently healthy adults between 18 and 64 years of age should accumulate at least 150 minutes of moderate to vigorous-intensity aerobic physical activity per week in bouts of 10 minutes or more. It is also beneficial to add muscle and bone-straightening activities using major muscle groups at least 2 days per week' [48].

From this perspective, the unhealthy habit can be modified positively through brief interventions based on education [49,50]. The patient should be given a full explanation of the mechanisms of exercise, including the importance of balanced training sessions, rest periods, and the negative effects of overtraining on health [47].

10.3.2 Motivational Interviewing

Motivational interviewing is a technique for increasing motivation to change [51]. It consists of four processes: (i) *engaging* in a working relationship based on trust and respect; (ii) *focusing* on the desired goal; (iii) *evoking* the individual's motivations for change; and (iv) *planning* a specific strategy for reaching the next step [52]. Therapists try to determine the person's stage of change (i.e., contemplation, preparation, or action) so that they can adopt the right therapeutic tool to help the patient to move towards the next stage (e.g., from contemplation to preparation) [52]. A study conducted by Dunn et al. in 2001 demonstrated that motivational interviewing is successful in inducing and maintaining positive outcomes in individuals with behavioural dependencies [53].

10.3.3 Cognitive–Behavioural Therapy

Cognitive–behavioural therapy (CBT) promotes the development of personal coping strategies to enable a person to change unhelpful patterns in cognitions (i.e., thoughts, beliefs, and attitudes), behaviours (e.g., unhealthy habits or addictions), and emotions (e.g., rage, anxiety, depression) [54–56]. It is regarded as the first-line treatment for other addictive behaviours, such as gambling [57], hypersexual disorder [58], kleptomania [59], and compulsive buying [60], but has also produced positive outcomes in patients with EA [61]. The primary objective is to change the patient's attitudes towards physical activity. The therapist might identify attitudes, beliefs, and emotions that have led the patient to engage in addictive exercise [62]. This type of addiction is often accompanied by low self-esteem, distorted body image, and perfectionist tendencies [63]. Developing self-esteem involves allowing the individual to build a self-concept that is not connected either to their appearance or to social approval [63]. The patient must identify why exercise is so rewarding in terms of self-esteem, and then learn alternative ways to obtain the same rewards. In 2003, Adams et al. drew up the following therapeutic intervention guidelines for clinicians, with a focus on cognitive processing and behavioural management: (i) identify and interrupt the compulsive behaviour through supportive individual psychotherapy; (ii) engage the patient in understanding the health benefits and importance of moderation; (iii) empower the patient to develop a self-management strategy; (iv) understand the organization of the patient's defence structure and how they are coping with the addictive personality; (v) increase the tolerance of the patient in adapting to or accommodating the compulsion through modification of their psychological defences and acceptance and understanding of their responses to the gaining of control and appropriate self-management skills; (vi) unlink the compulsion- and process-specific triggers related to the EA; (vii) rebuild the coping behaviours and enhance the patient's support system with regard to exercise [44]. CBT has also been associated with *contingency management*, with good outcomes [64]. Patients were tested regularly to check that they were not engaging in harmful behaviour; they received positive reinforcement if they passed the test, but were penalized if they failed [64]. The association of the rewarding of positive behaviour with CBT-based cognitive restructuring and increasing coping skills was found to be highly effective [65].

10.3.4 Mindfulness-Based Psychotherapy

Mindfulness-based cognitive–behavioural therapy (MCBT) uses CBT in conjunction with mindfulness meditation [66]. Through CBT the patient is educated about their addictive behaviour. Mindfulness meditation focuses on becoming aware of all incoming thoughts and feelings and accepting them without reacting to them [67]. The aim of this process, known as 'decentring', is to disengage from all the negative emotions that can arise when one is reacting to negative thinking patterns [68]. This therapy has been widely used to treat substance use disorders [69]: Shonin et al. recently suggested that this approach may have psychotherapeutic value for countering the negative thoughts that result from a behavioural addiction [70]. This interesting therapeutic approach needs to be further investigated with larger samples and systematic studies.

10.4 Pharmacological Interventions

The pharmacological treatment of behavioural addictions is currently based only on empirical assessments and clinical characteristics similar to those of obsessive-compulsive disorder (OCD) and impulsive-compulsive spectrum disorders [71]. In addition, neuropsychological tests have revealed that behavioural and substance-related addictions share similar anomalies in complex executive functions, such as planning, mood modulation, attention, elaboration of problem-solving strategies, exaggerated reward sensitivity, and maintenance of abnormal and increased levels of excitation and deficient self-control [72]. Different options have been investigated, including antidepressants, mood stabilizers, opioid antagonists, glutamatergic modulators, and antipsychotics, all of which have been shown to be effective in reducing symptoms and controlling cravings [73]. There have been only a few studies of the use of pharmacological treatments in EA. However, other behavioural addictions have been successfully treated with medications, leading to the production of guidelines which, after further investigations, might be applied to EA as well.

10.4.1 Selective Serotonin Reuptake Inhibitors

Selective serotonin reuptake inhibitors (SSRIs) seem to play an important role in the treatment of behavioural addictions due to their action on the serotoninergic system. Studies of their use in pathological gambling have shown a good response to fluvoxamine [74–76], paroxetine [77], citalopram [78], and escitalopram [79], characterized by increased quality of life and a general improvement in compulsive symptoms. Similar results have been reported for compulsive shopping [80,81], sex addiction [82–84], and video-game cravings [85,86].

10.4.2 Naltrexone

Naltrexone is an opioid μ-receptor antagonist that has a role in modulating dopaminergic transmission in the mesolimbic area, and is commonly used in the treatment of alcohol and opioid dependence [87]. It has shown good outcomes in patients characterized by marked impulsive traits, but its use is limited by the risk of severe liver toxicity [88]. Positive results have been reported in the treatment of pathological gambling [89] and compulsive shopping [90,91], as well as in technology addiction, where naltrexone reduced compulsive searching for online pornography [92].

10.4.3 Glutamatergic Modulators

Neurochemical and genetic evidence suggests that glutamate deregulation may contribute to the exacerbation of compulsive symptoms [93], and improved glutamatergic tone in the nucleus accumbens has been associated with a reduction in reward-seeking behaviour in addiction [73]. N-acetylcysteine has shown some degree of efficacy in gambling disorder [94], and memantine appears to reduce impulsive behaviours in pathological shopping [95].

10.4.4 Mood Stabilizers

Only a few data are available on the effectiveness of mood stabilizers such as lithium salts, carbamazepine, valproate, topiramate, and gabapentin. The similarities between impulsive behaviours and the manic phases of bipolar disorder suggested their potential use in non-drug addictions [96]. Lithium salts and topiramate monotherapy showed good results in gambling disorder [97,98]. Mood stabilizers with GABAergic inhibitory activity on the frontal lobes (i.e., valproate, lamotrigine, gabapentin, pregabalin, topiramate, and vigabatrin) have been proposed as a treatment for sex addiction, but to date the results have been inconclusive [71].

10.4.5 Antipsychotics

Atypical antipsychotics have been used to enhance the effects of serotonin reuptake inhibitors (SRIs) and SSRIs in treatment-resistant obsessive-compulsive disorder. For this reason, some studies have evaluated their use in the treatment of behavioural addictions [74]. In particular, olanzapine was reported to be useful in video-poker addiction [99], and quetiapine has been used to treat a complex case of overtraining. The latter involved a patient who had been diagnosed with bipolar I disorder, compulsive buying, and EA. After 12 weeks of treatment the behavioural symptoms had significantly improved, and after 24 weeks they had completely resolved. The patient's score on the Exercise Addiction Inventory (EAI) had decreased from 28 at admission to 12 after the treatment [100]. Further studies are needed on the potential use of these medications for behavioural addictions, and specifically for EA.

10.5 Conclusion

As concepts such as fitspiration take hold, boosted by media and social network images, physical activity – even when excessive or counterproductive – is accepted rather than stigmatized in today's society. Therefore EA is probably the most 'hidden' behavioural addiction. As it may become maladaptive and health-threatening, its prompt recognition and treatment may be very challenging both for healthcare professionals and for the family and friends of the affected person. The lack of guidance and literature on the topic may further complicate diagnosis and treatment. Although EA is not included in the DSM-5, it is mandatory to inform clinicians about it, as well as other healthcare providers, such as psychotherapists and physiotherapists, to enable them to recognize early signs of this addiction and prevent injuries or other serious effects on physical or mental health. This chapter has presented a synopsis of the treatment of EA, as well as information about the aetiological basis of the disorder, and a compendium of psychological and pharmacological interventions.

EA is a multifactorial disorder in which internal factors (personality traits and negative experiences) and external factors (environment and social values) act together during its onset, development, and maintenance. Therefore the clinical approach should address every aspect of the patient's suffering. The beneficial effects of sports should be presented with caution by media and professionals, highlighting the importance of a well-designed fitness routine with planned rest periods, which are essential to allow the body to recover properly. Society plays a key role here. Parents, teachers, health educators, coaches, fitness instructors, and other professionals involved must cooperate in identifying and intervening when signs of dysfunctional exercise occur [46]. People who exercise excessively should be evaluated and, depending on the symptom severity, comorbidities, and other associated addictions, offered treatment [31]. A specific assessment of whether EA is primary or secondary to another specific condition (e.g., eating disorders) should be undertaken in order to guide therapy. Particular attention should be given to a possible link between EA and the use of IPEDs and other medical or non-medical products, in order to minimize the associated health risks [18,36]. Psychotherapy appears to be the first-line treatment for EA. The use of medication should be limited to selected cases that are characterized by severe symptoms or complicated by other comorbidities. In this case, the use of psychotropic drugs may help to reduce the negative feelings associated with the urge to exercise, and allow the patient to remain more focused on therapy. Further studies involving larger samples are required in order to gain a broader understanding of this subject.

References

1   Bouchard C, Shephard RJ, Stephens T. *Physical Activity, Fitness, and Health: International Proceedings and Consensus Statement*. Human Kinetics Publishers, 1994.

2   Szabo A. The impact of exercise deprivation on well-being of habitual exercisers. *Aust J Sci Med Sport* 1995; 27: 68–75.

3   Szabo A. Studying the psychological impact of exercise deprivation: are experimental studies hopeless? *J Sport Behav* 1998; 21: 139–47.

4   Szabo A. Physical activity as a source of psychological dysfunction. In: Biddle SJ, Fox KR, Boutcher SH, eds. *Physical Activity and Psychological Well-Being*. Routledge, 2000: 130–53.

5   Smith LL. Overtraining, excessive exercise, and altered immunity. *Sports Med* 2003; 33: 347–64.

6   Morgan WP. Negative addiction in runners. *Phys Sportsmed* 1979; 7: 57–70.

7   Hailey BJ, Bailey LA. Negative addiction in runners: a quantitative approach. *J Sport Behav* 1982; 5:150–4.

8 Hausenblas HA, Downs DS. Relationship among sex, imagery, and exercise dependence symptoms. *Psychol Addict Behav* 2002; 16: 169–72.

9 Veale DMW. Exercise dependence. *Br J Addict* 1987; 82: 735–40.

10 Hausenblas HA, Downs DS. How much is too much? The development and validation of the Exercise Dependence Scale. *Psychol Health* 2002; 17: 387–404.

11 Downs DS, Hausenblas HA, Nigg CR. Factorial validity and psychometric examination of the Exercise Dependence Scale-Revised. *Meas Phys Educ Exerc Sci* 2004; 8: 183–201.

12 Haasova M, Warren FC, Ussher M et al. The acute effects of physical activity on cigarette cravings: systematic review and meta-analysis with individual participant data. *Addiction* 2013; 108: 26–37.

13 Read JP, Brown, R. The role of physical exercise in alcoholism treatment and recovery. *Prof Psychol Res Pr* 2003; 34: 49–56.

14 Manthou E, Georgakouli K, Fatouros I et al. Role of exercise in the treatment of alcohol use disorders. *Biomed Rep* 2016; 4: 535–45.

15 Lichtenstein MB, Emborg B, Hemmingsen SD, Hansen NB. Is exercise addiction in fitness centers a socially accepted behavior? *Addict Behav Rep* 2017; 6: 102–5.

16 Mabe AG, Forney KJ, Keel PK. Do you like my photo? Facebook use maintains eating disorder risk. *Int J Eat Disord* 2014; 47: 516–23.

17 Meier EP, Gray J. Facebook photo activity associated with body image disturbance in adolescent girls. *Cyberpsychol Behav Soc Netw* 2014; 17: 199–206.

18 Corazza O, Simonato P, Demetrovics Z et al. The emergence of exercise addiction, body dysmorphic disorder, and other image-related psychopathological correlates in fitness settings: a cross sectional study. *PLoS ONE* 2019; 14: e0213060.

19 Holland G, Tiggemann M. A systematic review of the impact of the use of social networking sites on body image and disordered eating outcomes. *Body Image* 2016; 17: 100–10.

20 Holland G, Tiggemann M. "Strong beats skinny every time": disordered eating and compulsive exercise in women who post fitspiration on Instagram. *Int J Eat Disord* 2017; 50: 76–9.

21 Brown I. A theoretical model of the behavioural addictions—applied to offending. In: Hodge JE, McMurran M, Hollins CR, eds. *Addicted to Crime?* John Wiley & Sons, 1997: 13–65.

22 Andreassen CS, Griffiths MD, Gjertsen SR et al. The relationships between behavioral addictions and the five-factor model of personality. *J Behav Addict* 2013; 2: 90–9.

23 Griffiths MD, Szabo A, Terry A. The Exercise Addiction Inventory: a quick and easy screening tool for health practitioners. *Br J Sports Med* 2005; 39: e30.

24 Lichtenstein MB, Emborg B, Daugaard Hemmingsen S, Hansen NB. Is exercise addiction in fitness centers a socially accepted behavior? *Addict Behav Rep* 2017; 6: 102–5.

25 Lichtenstein MB, Christiansen E, Elklit A, Bilenberg N, Støving RK. Exercise addiction: a study of eating disorder symptoms, quality of life, personality traits and attachment styles. *Psychiatry Res* 2014; 357: 410–16.

26 Anandkumar S, Manivasagam M, Kee VTS, Meyding-Lamade U. Effect of physical therapy management of nonspecific low back pain with exercise addiction behaviors: a case series. *Physiother Theory Pract* 2018; 34: 316–28.

27 Schwellnus M, Soligard T, Alonso JM et al. How much is too much? (Part 2) International Olympic Committee consensus statement on load in sport and risk of illness. *Br J Sports Med* 2016; 357: 1043–52.

28 De Souza MJ, Nattiv A, Joy E et al. 2014 Female Athlete Triad Coalition Consensus Statement on Treatment and Return to Play of the Female Athlete Triad: 1st International Conference held in San Francisco, California, May 2012 and 2nd International Conference held in Indianapolis, Indiana, May 2013. *Br J Sports Med* 2014; 48: 289.

29 Meeusen R, Duclos M, Foster C et al. Prevention, diagnosis, and treatment of the overtraining syndrome: joint consensus statement of the European College of Sport Science and the American College of Sports Medicine. *Med Sci Sports Exerc* 2013; 45: 186–205.

30 Hausenblas HA, Schreiber K, Smoliga JM, Addiction to exercise. *BMJ* 2017; 357: j1745.

31 Weinstein A, Maayan G, Weinstein Y. A study on the relationship between compulsive exercise, depression and anxiety. *J Behav Addict* 2015; 4: 315–18.

32 Antunes HK, Leite GS, Lee KS et al. Exercise deprivation increases negative mood in exercise-addicted subjects and modifies their biochemical markers. *Physiol Behav* 2016; 357: 182–90.

33 Pope Jnr HG, Katz DL, Champoux R. Anabolic-androgenic steroid use among 1,010 college men. *Phys Sportsmed* 1988; 16: 75–81.

34 Corazza O, Demetrovics Z, van den Brink W, Schifano F. 'Legal highs' an inappropriate term for 'Novel Psychoactive Drugs' in drug prevention and scientific debate. *Int J Drug Policy* 2013; 24: 82–3.

35 Van Hout MC. SMART: an Internet study of users' experiences of synthetic tanning. *Perform Enhanc Health* 2014; 3: 3–14.

36 Mooney R, R Simonato P, Ruparelia R et al. The use of supplements and performance and image enhancing drugs in fitness settings: an exploratory cross-sectional investigation in the United Kingdom. *Hum Psychopharmacol* 2017; 32: e2619.

37 Freimuth M, Moniz S, Kim SR. Clarifying exercise addiction: differential diagnosis, co-occurring disorders, and phases of addiction. *Int J Environ Res Public Health* 2011; 8: 4069–81.

38 Bruno A, Quattrone D, Scimeca G et al. Unraveling exercise addiction: the role of narcissism and self-esteem. *J Addict* 2014; 2014: 987841.

39 Levallius J, Collin C, Birgegård A. Now you see it, now you don't: compulsive exercise in adolescents with an eating disorder. *J Eat Disord* 2017; 5: 9.

40 Rocks T, Pelly F, Slater G, Martin LA. Prevalence of exercise addiction symptomology and disordered eating in Australian students studying nutrition and dietetics. *J Acad Nutr Diet* 2017; 117: 1628–36.

41 Klein DA, Bennett AS, Schebendach J et al. Exercise "addiction" in anorexia nervosa: model development and pilot data. *CNS Spectr* 2004, 9: 531–7.

42 Veale DMW. Does primary exercise dependence really exist? In: Annet J, Cripps B, Steinberg H, eds. *Exercise Addiction: Motivation for Participation in Sport and Exercise*. British Psychological Society, 1995: 71–5.

43 Adams J, Kirkby RJ. Exercise dependence and overtraining: the psychological and physiological consequences of excessive exercise. *Res Sports Med* 2001; 10: 199–222.

44 Adams JM, Miller TW, Kraus RF. Exercise dependence: diagnostic and therapeutic issues for patients in psychotherapy. *J Contemp Psychother* 2003; 33: 93–107.

45 Blaydon MJ, Lindner KJ, Kerr JH. Metamotivational characteristics of eating-disordered and exercise-dependent triathletes: an application of reversal theory. *Psychol Sport Exerc* 2004; 3: 223–36.

46 Berczik K, Szabó A, Griffiths MD et al. Exercise addiction: symptoms, diagnosis, epidemiology, and etiology. *Subst Use Misuse* 2002; 47: 403–17.

47 Adams J, Kirkby RJ. Excessive exercise as an addiction: a review. *Addict Res Theory* 2002; 10: 415–37.

48 Canadian Society for Exercise Physiology. *Make Your Whole Day Matter: The Canadian 24-Hour Movement Guidelines for Adults (18-64 years)*. Canadian Society for Exercise Physiology, 2016. www.csepguidelines.ca/adults-18-64

49 Bogers RP, van Assema P, Brug J, Kester ADM, Dagnelie PC. Psychosocial predictors of increases in fruit and vegetable consumption. *Am J Health Behav* 2007; 31: 135–45.

50 Seligman HK, Wallace AS, DeWalt DA et al. Facilitating behavior change with low-literacy patient education materials. *Am J Health Behav* 2007; 31: S69–78.

51 Miller WR, Rollnick S. *Motivational Interviewing: Preparing People for Change*, 2nd ed. The Guilford Press, 2002.

52 Miller WR, Rollnick S. *Motivational Interviewing: Preparing People to Change Addictive Behavior*. The Guilford Press, 1991.

53 Dunn C, Deroo L, Rivara FP. The use of brief interventions adapted from motivational interviewing across behavioral domains: a systematic review. *Addiction* 2001; 96: 1725–42.

54 Beck JS. *Cognitive Behavior Therapy: Basics and Beyond*, 2nd ed. The Guilford Press, 2011.

55 Field TA, Beeson ET, Jones LK. The new ABCs: a practitioner's guide to neuroscience-informed cognitive-behavior therapy. *J Ment Health Couns* 2015; 37: 206–20.

56 Benjamin CL, Puleo CM, Settipani CA et al. History of cognitive-behavioral therapy (CBT) in youth. *Child Adolesc Psychiatr Clin N Am* 2011; 20: 179–89.

57 Cowlishaw S, Merkouris S, Dowling N et al. Psychological therapies for pathological and problem gambling. *Cochrane Database Syst Rev* 2012; 11: CD008937.

58 Hook JN, Reid RC, Penberthy JK, Davis DE, Jennings DJ 2nd. Methodological review of treatments for nonparaphilic hypersexual behavior. *J Sex Marital Ther* 2014; 40: 294–308.

59 Christianini AR, Conti MA, Hearst N et al. Treating kleptomania: cross-cultural adaptation of the Kleptomania Symptom Assessment Scale and assessment of an outpatient program. *Compr Psychiatry* 2015; 56: 289–94.

60 Lourenço Leite P, Pereira VM, Nardi AE, Silva AC. Psychotherapy for compulsive buying disorder: a systematic review. *Psychiatry Res* 2014; 219: 411–19.

61 Wichmann S, Martin DR. Exercise excess: treating patients addicted to fitness. *Phys Sportsmed* 1992; 20: 193–200.

62 Fisher LA, Wrisberg CA. A "positive psychology" of athletic training. *Athl Ther Today* 2004; 9: 58–9.

63 Cumella E. The heavy weight of exercise addiction. *Behav Health Manag* 2005; 25: 26–31.

64 Moeller FG, Schmitz JM, Steinberg JL et al. Citalopram combined with behavioral therapy reduces cocaine use: a double-blind, placebo-controlled trial. *Am J Drug Alcohol Abuse* 2007; 33: 367–78.

65 Adams J. Understanding exercise dependence. *J Contemp Psychother* 2009, 39: 231–40.

66 Manicavasgar V, Parker G, Perich, T. Mindfulness-based cognitive therapy vs. cognitive behaviour therapy as a treatment for non-melancholic depression. *J Affect Disord* 2011; 130: 138–44.

67 Hofmann SG, Sawyer AT, Fang A. The empirical status of the "new wave" of cognitive behavioral therapy. *Psychiatr Clin N Am* 2010; 33: 701–10.

68 Hayes SC, Villatte M, Levin M, Hildebrandt M. Open, aware, and active: contextual approaches as an emerging trend in the behavioral and cognitive therapies. *Annu Rev Clin Psychol* 2011; 7: 141–68.

69 Zgierska A, Rabago D, Chawla N et al. Mindfulness meditation for substance use disorders: a systematic review. *Subst Abus* 2009; 30: 266–94.

70 Shonin E, Van Gordon W, Griffiths MD. Buddhist philosophy for the treatment of problem gambling. *J Behav Addict* 2013; 2: 63–71.

71 Marazziti D. *Farmacoterapia Clinica*, 5th ed. Fioriti, 2013.

72 Goldstein RZ, Volkow ND. Drug addiction and its underlying neurobiological basis: neuroimaging evidence for the involvement of the frontal cortex. *Am J Psychiatry* 2002; 159: 1642–52.

73 Marazziti D, Presta S, Baroni S, Silvestri S, Dell'Osso L. Behavioral addictions: a novel challenge for psychopharmacology. *CNS Spectr* 2014; 19: 486–95.

74 Hollander E, DeCaria CM, Mari E. Short-term single-blind fluvoxamine treatment of pathological gambling. *Am J Psychiatry* 1998; 155: 1781–3.

75 Hollander E, DeCaria CM, Finkell JN et al. A randomized double-blind fluvoxamine/placebo crossover trial in pathologic gambling. *Biol Psychiatry* 2000; 47: 813–17.

76 Blanco C, Petkova E, Ibanez A, Saiz-Ruiz J. A pilot placebo-controlled study of fluvoxamine for pathological gambling. *Ann Clin Psychiatry* 2002; 14: 9–15.

77 Kim SW, Grant JE, Adson DE, Shin YC, Zaninelli R. A double-blind placebo-controlled study of the efficacy and safety of paroxetine in the treatment of pathological gambling. *J Clin Psychiatry* 2002; 63: 501–7.

78 Zimmerman M, Breen RB, Posternak MA. An open-label study of citalopram in the treatment of pathological gambling. *J Clin Psychiatry* 2002; 63: 44–8.

79 Black DW, Shaw M, Forbush KT, Allen J. An open-label trial of escitalopram in the treatment of pathological gambling. *Clin Neuropharmacol* 2007; 30: 206–12.

80 McElroy SL, Satlin A, Pope HG, Keck PE, Hudson J. Treatment of compulsive shopping with antidepressants: a report of three cases. *Ann Clin Psychiatry* 1991; 3: 199–204.

81 McElroy SL, Keck PE Jr, Pope HG Jr, Smith JM, Strakowski SM. Compulsive buying: a report on 20 cases. *J Clin Psychiatry* 1994; 55: 242–8.

82 Emmanuel NP, Lydiard RB, Ballenger JC. Fluoxetine treatment of voyeurism. *Am J Psychiatry* 1991; 148: 950.

83 Stein DJ, Hollander E, Anthony DT et al. Serotonergic medications for sexual obsessions, sexual addiction, and paraphilias. *J Clin Psychiatry* 1992; 53: 267–71.

84 Fedoroff JP. Serotonergic drug treatment of deviant sexual interests. *Ann Sex Res* 1993; 6: 105–21.

85 Sattar P, Ramaswamy S. Internet gaming addiction. *Can J Psychiatry* 2004; 49: 869–70.

86 Dell'Osso B, Altamura AC, Hadley SJ, Baker BR, Hollander E. An open-label trial of escitalopram in the treatment of impulsive-compulsive internet usage disorder. *Eur Neuropsychopharmacol* 2006; 16: S82–3.

87 American Society of Health-System Pharmacists. *Naltrexone.* Drugs.com, 2017. www.drugs.com/monograph/naltrexone.html

88 Kim SW, Grant JE, Adson DE, Shin YC. Double-blind naltrexone and placebo comparison study in the treatment of pathological gambling. *Biol Psychiatry* 2001; 49: 914–21.

89 Grant JE, Potenza MN, Hollander E et al. Multicenter investigation of the opioid antagonist nalmefene in the treatment of pathological gambling. *Am J Psychiatry* 2006; 163: 303–12.

90 Bullock K, Koran L. Psychopharmacology of compulsive buying. *Drugs Today (Barc)* 2003; 39: 695–700.

91 Guzman CS, Filomensky T, Tavares H. Compulsive buying treatment with topiramate: a case report. *Braz J Psychiatry* 2007; 29: 383–4.

92 Bostwick JM, Bucci A. Internet sex addiction treated with naltrexone. *Mayo Clin Proc* 2008; 83: 226–30.

93 Pittenger C. Glutamate modulators in the treatment of obsessive-compulsive disorder. *Psychiatr Ann* 2015; 45: 308–15.

94 Grant JE, Kim SW, Odlaug BL. N-acetyl cysteine, a glutamate modulating agent, in the treatment of pathological gambling: a pilot study. *Biol Psychiatry* 2007; 62: 652–7.

95 Grant JE, Odlaug BL, Mooney M, O'Brien R, Kim SW. Open-label pilot study of memantine in the treatment of compulsive buying. *Ann Clin Psychiatry* 2012; 24: 119–26.

96 McElroy SL, Pope HG, Keck PE et al. Are impulse control disorders related to bipolar disorder? *Compr Psychiatry* 1996; 37: 229–40.

97 Pallanti S, Quercioli L, Sood E, Hollander E. Lithium and valproate treatment of pathological gambling: a randomized single-blind study. *J Clin Psychiatry* 2002; 63: 559–66.

98 Dannon PN, Lowengrub K, Gonopolski Y, Musin E, Kotler M. Topiramate versus fluvoxamine in the treatment of pathological gambling: a randomized, blind-rater, comparison study. *Clin Neuropharmacol* 2005; 28: 6–10.

99 Fong T, Kalechstein A, Bernhard B, Rosenthal R, Rugle LA. A double-blind, placebo-controlled trial of olanzapine for the treatment of video poker pathological gamblers. *Pharmacol Biochem Behav* 2008; 89: 298–303.

100 Di Nicola M, Martinotti G, Mazza M et al. Quetiapine as add-on treatment for bipolar I disorder with comorbid compulsive buying and physical exercise addiction. *Prog Neuropsychopharmacol Biol Psychiatry* 2010; 34: 713–14.

Chapter 11

Being Versus Appearing: Two Sides of the Same Coin?

A Case Report

Artemisa Rocha Dores and Pedro Morgado

11.1 Introduction

We are living in an era in which the personal value of individuals seems to be determined more by what they look like than by their personal qualities and skills [1]. For some people this misconception about their value can become a trap in which reality is blurred. This may affect personal goals and the commitment to them, and ultimately can harm mental health [2–6]. Appearance and body image may become the main focus of thoughts and actions, leading to physical, psychological, and social suffering, about which people may or may not have insight [7].

This chapter presents the case of a 32-year-old man, who attended for a psychiatric consultation because of his belief that his current medication was preventing him from gaining the weight needed to achieve the body shape he desired. At that time he believed that his body was not sufficiently muscled, as he considered that it was essential for him to have a muscular physique if he was to return to his previous professional activity. He was practising about 5 hours of weight training daily, 7 days a week, to achieve his goal, and thus fulfilled the criteria for body dysmorphic disorder (BDD) [7]. The development of that diagnosis had been insidious, and was preceded by a history of bipolar disorder and anxiety symptomatology. A treatment plan that combined psychotropic medications and psychotherapy was found to be effective in reducing his symptoms.

11.2 Case Report

J, a 32-year-old man, had started to attend regular psychiatric follow-up sessions at the age of 19 years, after he had developed symptoms of depression. He grew up in a nuclear family consisting of his father, mother, and three brothers. He showed normal psychomotor development, and attended school regularly, completing 12 years of formal education. He described himself as heterosexual, and had no known lasting relationships.

The diagnosis at that time was major depressive disorder, and J had been prescribed sertraline 100 mg and diazepam 5 mg. The depressive condition had a strong somatic component and intense ideation with hypochondriac content. J experienced intense suffering and was emotionally exuberant. He did not receive psychotherapy, due to a lack of mental health resources in the National Health Service or private funds for such treatment. After 3 months, J experienced remission of his symptoms, and he stopped the medication after 12 months of treatment.

New depressive episodes occurred when J was 23 years old, and 2 years later. No information is available about the treatment he was given at that time. During that period he had several short-term jobs in the catering industry.

At the age of 28 years, he presented with an episode characterized by increased psychomotor activity and disinhibition, with dysphoric humour that was treated as a hypomanic episode. At that time he was unemployed. He was prescribed quetiapine 800 mg/day, which resulted in an improvement in his mood, and a diagnosis of bipolar II disorder was then established.

At the age of 29 years, J enrolled on a flight attendant course, and he started going to the gym regularly, initially for 3 days a week. His mood was euthymic, and he stopped going to the psychiatric sessions which he had been attending for the last year. At that time, he only kept the medication prescribed by his family doctor. He worked as a flight attendant in an aviation company, in a replacement position, for 6 months. He then became unemployed, and his level of physical exercise increased. He started practising weight training for 3–5 hours every day of the week. He also started taking anabolic steroids regularly, with the aim of increasing his muscle mass. Paradoxically, he had no particular concerns about diet.

At the age of 32, J returned for a psychiatric consultation. At that time he was practising about 5 hours of weight training every day of the week, including Sundays. He had not been employed regularly for 2 years, and was taking quetiapine 800 mg/day. He believed that his body was not sufficiently muscular, and his aim was to increase his muscle mass so that he could return to work for an airline. Exercise and investment in body image were his main personal motivations. He no longer associated with his former group of friends because he wanted to avoid going out for meals with them (so that he could control his food intake) or socializing with them at night (so that he could avoid drinking). He reported feelings of irritability when he missed a training session, and also sporadic sexual encounters with a friend from the gym.

At that time he wanted to reduce his medication, as he believed that the quetiapine was preventing him from reaching the target weight that he considered necessary to achieve his desired body shape. At the same consultation he presented with depressed mood and dysmorphophobia. He also complained of severe initial insomnia and intense anxiety. He was prescribed quetiapine 400 mg/day, venlafaxine 150 mg/day, and lorazepam 2.5 mg/day. To improve his depressed mood and insomnia, the medication was adjusted 4 weeks later by the addition of mirtazapine 15 mg/day. Despite having a body mass index (BMI) of 27.04 kg m^2 (based on a body weight of 80 kg and height of 1.72 m), he still complained about being underweight and he continued to maintain the same intensity of training.

J experienced an improvement in mood after 8 weeks of treatment. However, he maintained the dysmorphophobic ideation that his body weight was too low and that his body was insufficiently muscular. A diagnosis of BDD was established. The quetiapine dose was adjusted to 200 mg/day, and he began to attend psychotherapy sessions.

11.3 Therapeutic Interventions and Outcomes

The first phase of psychotherapy aimed to increase J's awareness of the problem of excessive exercise and its consequences for both his health and the other areas of his life. The second phase sought to define realistic goals with him, and to work on cognitions related to dysmorphophobia.

After 4 months of psychotherapeutic follow-up, J maintained a euthymic mood. He experienced periods of anxiety related to his dysmorphophobic beliefs. He engaged in 4 hours of exercise each day and exhibited intense dysfunctionality, as he was neither working nor participating in social activities, and he kept to his goal of increasing muscle mass and body weight.

Against this background, cognitions related to self-image and self-esteem were worked on. A plan with more realistic objectives that were adjusted to J's needs was drawn up with him. Employment issues were addressed with the specific aims of helping him to achieve success in the catering industry and deal with the feelings of failure associated with his job as a flight attendant.

After 8 months, J had reduced his attendance at the gym from 7 days per week to 5 days per week. He maintained intense dysmorphophobia about his body weight, which remained at 82 kg. His medication was again adjusted, to quetiapine 200 mg/day, mirtazapine 30 mg/day, lorazepam 2.5 mg/day, and clomipramine 150 mg/day.

After 12 months of treatment, J had reduced his gym attendance to 4 days per week, training for about 3 hours per day. He maintained his dysmorphophobic ideation, and his weight increased slightly, to 83 kg. His medication regime remained unchanged.

11.4 Discussion

BDD is classified under 'Obsessive-Compulsive and Related Disorders' in DSM-5, along with obsessive-compulsive disorder and several other conditions [7]. BDD is a mental health disorder in which the affected person is troubled by or cannot stop thinking about one or more perceived defects or flaws in their appearance, which tend to be minor or cannot even be detected by other people. As a result, people with BDD may feel embarrassed, ashamed, and anxious, and avoid many social situations. The perceived flaws and the repetitive behaviours associated with them (e.g., repeatedly checking the mirror, grooming, or seeking reassurance from others) may cause significant distress, which affects the person's ability to function adequately in daily life. These perceptions cause clinically significant distress or impairment in important areas of functioning, for which treatment is required [7]. This was the case for J, who as described earlier presented with impairment of daily functioning that had an impact on several life domains, including social aspects (e.g., restricted interactions with others) and occupational aspects (e.g., unemployment). According to him, the reduction in social interactions was due not to a desire to avoid his friends, but rather to avoid the caloric gain associated with food and alcohol consumption that would occur if he went out with them.

Although individuals with BDD tend to resort to numerous treatments in an attempt to overcome or 'fix' perceived flaws in their appearance, they often do not seek treatment for BDD itself, despite the dysfunctionality that they (and, indirectly, their family) experience as a result of this constellation of signs and symptoms [8]. In the case of J, psychiatric treatment was not sought as a way to control or resolve the manifestations of BDD, as he believed that the medication he was taking for other symptoms at that time was preventing him from achieving his 'ideal' body weight and musculature.

The specific aetiology and pathophysiology of BDD are still not known in detail. This disorder may result from a combination of factors that increase the risk of its development, such as family history of the disorder, negative evaluations or experiences of one's body or self-image, and age (BDD is most common among teenagers and young adults). Attempts to integrate some of these possible contributory factors within the framework of conceptual theories and models have been identified (for a review, see [9]). For example, Feusner et al. [10] developed a preliminary and overarching model of the aetiological and pathophysiological processes that appear to contribute to the development and maintenance of BDD. It includes biological and genetic susceptibility, adverse life events, cognitive distortions, and learned behaviour. In addition, the well-known cognitive–behavioural therapy (CBT) models proposed by Veale [11], and more recently by Wilhelm et al. [12], integrate biological, psychological, and sociocultural factors. In the case of J, the desired professional activity, in which body image was valued, combined with negative life experiences such as unemployment, could have created real or imaginary pressure to achieve a 'perfect' body.

In J's case we observed that, in order to obtain the 'perfect' body that he perceived as the key to success, he became increasingly involved in physical exercise (i.e., weight training) and the (mis)use of performance- and image-enhancing drugs (i.e., anabolic steroids) [1,13]. He also experienced excessive unwanted thoughts that became difficult to control and were very time-consuming. As a result of this scenario, he found himself caught in a vicious cycle in which perfection was never achieved.

It has been recognized that compensating behaviours can potentially become addictive [14,15]. These behaviours can occur excessively, becoming compulsive and problematic for some individuals, with harmful physical, financial, and social consequences [16,17]. The exercise addiction (EA) construct is the most frequently encountered compulsive behaviour, but it is still controversial. There is a need for reliable theory-driven research and clinical evidence, which may allow us to differentiate regular and excessive exercising from a behavioural addiction. With regard to Griffiths' six components of addiction (salience, mood modification, tolerance, withdrawal symptoms, conflict, and relapse), J exhibited four of the components, namely salience, tolerance, withdrawal, and conflict [14,15,18]. This distinguished the present case from those in which the individuals are simply highly committed to exercising.

In addition to the contributory factors already mentioned, it is possible that BDD might have been triggered by the presence of another mental health disorder, and indeed J had a history of bipolar II disorder.

BDD treatment might include psychological treatment, psychotherapy, and/or medication. The pharmacological approach, such as the use of selective serotonin reuptake inhibitors (SSRIs), and psychological or psychotherapeutic approaches, namely the use of CBT alone or in combination, are all empirically based treatments [19]. Several studies have shown that CBT is effective in reducing the severity and related symptoms (e.g., depression) of BDD [12,20,21]. In J's case, the use of psychotherapy and medication as a combined approach was only possible at a later stage in the progression of the disorder, due to lack of mental health resources in the National Health Service, but this combination proved to be effective.

The relationship between the different disorders presented in the case described in this chapter has been demonstrated in a recent study, which showed just such an association between EA, appearance anxiety, and BDD among a cohort of gym users. In addition, those authors highlighted the use of fitness products, including illicit drugs, as was also demonstrated in the case of J [4].

11.5 Main Lessons Learned

We always learn with our clients and patients. With J we learned a number of lessons. First, the age of onset could be different from the typically reported range, and therefore we must be alert to the emergence of this disorder at any age. Second, BDD was diagnosed in the context of a person suffering from a mood disorder (in this case bipolar II disorder) that appeared to be an aetiological factor. Third, it is possible to identify a set of very clear triggering factors. Finally, psychotherapeutic intervention is essential.

However, these disorders and conditions are difficult to treat. Even when a combination of treatments is used, it is possible that in some cases the symptoms will remit and in others they will remain, highlighting the need for further studies and new and innovative treatments.

References

1   Mooney R, Simonato P, Ruparelia R et al. The use of supplements and performance and image enhancing drugs in fitness settings: an exploratory cross-sectional investigation in the United Kingdom. *Hum Psychopharmacol* 2017; 32: e2619.

2   Altabe M, Thompson JK. Body image: a cognitive self-schema construct? *Cogn Ther Res* 1996; 20: 171–93.

3   Borchert J, Heinberg L. Gender schema and gender role discrepancy as correlates of body image. *J Psychol* 1996; 130: 547–59.

4   Corazza O, Simonato P, Demetrovics Z et al. The emergence of Exercise Addiction, Body Dysmorphic Disorder, and other image-related psychopathological correlates in fitness settings: a cross sectional study. *PLoS ONE* 2019; 14: e0213060.

5   Grant AM. An integrated model of goal-focused coaching: an evidence-based framework for teaching and practice. *Int Coach Psychol Rev* 2012; 7: 146–65.

6   Monteath SA, McCabe MP. The influence of societal factors on female body image. *J Soc Psychol* 1997; 137: 708–27.

7   American Psychiatric Association. *Diagnostic and Statistical Manual of Mental Disorders*, 5th ed. American Psychiatric Association, 2013.

8   Phillips KA, Dufresne RG Jr, Wilkel CS, Vittorio CC. Rate of body dysmorphic disorder in dermatology patients. *J Am Acad Dermatol* 2000; 42: 436–41.

9   Symons Downs D, MacIntyre RI, Heron KE. Exercise addiction and dependence. In: Anshel MH, Petruzzelo SJ, Labbé EE, eds. *APA Handbook of Sport and Exercise Psychology, Vol. 2. Exercise Psychology*. American Psychological Association, 2019: 589–604.

10   Feusner JD, Neziroglu F, Wilhelm S, Mancusi L, Bohon C. What causes BDD: research findings and a proposed model. *Psychiatr Ann* 2010; 40: 349–55.

11   Veale D. Advances in a cognitive behavioural model of body dysmorphic disorder. *Body Image* 2004; 1: 113–25.

12   Wilhelm S, Phillips KA, Steketee G. *Cognitive-Behavioral Therapy for Body Dysmorphic Disorder: A Treatment Manual*. The Guilford Press, 2013.

13   McVeigh J, Begley E. Anabolic steroids in the UK: an increasing issue for public health. *Drugs (Abingdon Engl)* 2016; 24: 278–85.

14 Griffiths MD. Exercise addiction: a case study. *Addict Res* 1997; 5: 161–8.

15 Griffiths MD. *Gambling and Gaming Addictions in Adolescence*. BPS Blackwell, 2002.

16 Szabo A. Studying the psychological impact of exercise deprivation: are experimental studies hopeless? *J Sport Behav* 1998; 21: 139–47.

17 Szabo A. Physical activity and psychological dysfunction. In: Biddle S, Fox K, Boutcher S, eds. *Physical Activity and Psychological Well-Being*. Routledge, 2000: 130–53.

18 Griffiths MD. Behavioural addiction: an issue for everybody? *J Workplace Learn* 1996; 8: 19–25.

19 Hartmann A, Greenberg J, Wilhelm S. *A Therapist's Guide for the Treatment of Body Dysmorphic Disorder*. International OCD Foundation, 2022. https://bdd.iocdf.org/professionals/therapists-guide-to-bdd-tx

20 Wilhelm S, Phillips KA, Didie E et al. Modular cognitive-behavioral therapy for body dysmorphic disorder: a randomized controlled trial. *Behav Ther* 2014; 45: 314–27.

21 Wilhelm S, Phillips KA, Fama JM, Greenberg JL, Steketee G. Modular cognitive-behavioral therapy for body dysmorphic disorder. *Behav Ther* 2011; 42: 624–33.

Chapter

12

Reducing Excessive Exercise Behaviour Using Online Cognitive–Behavioural Therapy

The Case of a Middle-Aged Adult

Merve Denizci Nazlıgül

12.1 Case Report

Luna, a 38-year-old divorced woman, has been working as a mathematician in Turkey. Her sister, who is 8 years older than her, is a gym teacher. Luna went to a boarding school during her secondary school years, and gained weight. When she came home for the holidays, her family members would call her names like 'Pudgy'. 'My family called me Pudgy with positive feelings because they loved the more sturdily built people in our culture. However, it was bothering me somewhat', she said. After this, Luna became obsessed with her weight and decided to follow a restricted diet. She subsequently reported that she had lost 10 kg.

With time, she became accustomed to carefully checking the ingredients of all the foods she consumed. In addition, she adopted a sugar- and carbohydrate-free diet for years. However, she also experienced feelings of losing control, which resulted in some sudden episodes of overeating. During these episodes she consumed abnormal amounts of food within minutes, with accompanying feelings of being unable to stop. She reported that she preferred certain types of foods when she engaged in binge-eating behaviour, and that she usually consumed sugary products such as ice cream or other desserts. She was most likely to engage in such eating behaviour when she was in distress. Then she began to feel guilt and regret about her binge-eating behaviour, and to get rid of those negative feelings she would exercise with increasing frequency and duration. Luna reported that exercise was a lifestyle for her. Her interest in sports began with mountain climbing during her college years, but after a serious injury she had to give up climbing, so she started running and CrossFit.

When Luna came to therapy, she was exercising for almost 2 hours per day, 6 days a week. In addition to this she did CrossFit, cycling, or running for nearly half an hour in the mornings, 2–3 days a week. She had been interested in marathons for a long time, and she now regularly joined training sessions for the races. She admitted that she preferred exercising to socializing with her friends. She also felt uneasy if her exercise was interrupted for any reason.

Luna had a boyfriend who was a member of the CrossFit club that she had joined. She reported that he criticized the appearance of her body and told her that she needed to exercise more. They broke up 4 months before she started therapy. After their relationship ended, Luna started to engage in extreme exercise to cope with her negative feelings. She mentioned that she could also overcome her feelings of loneliness through excessive watching of streaming services (e.g., Netflix) or by excessive eating. She had no psychiatric history, and was self-referred for individual psychotherapy.

12.2 Assessment and Case Conceptualization

Since the therapist and client did not live in the same city, the assessment and psychotherapy sessions were held online. All assessment measures and homework materials were sent by email. At the start of the treatment, Luna was asked to complete the Beck Depression Inventory (BDI) [1] and the Beck Anxiety Inventory (BAI) [2] so that her depressive and anxiety symptoms could be evaluated during the initial assessment interview. Her initial scores were 12 for the BDI (indicating mild depression) and 19 for the BAI (indicating moderate anxiety). In addition, she was asked to complete the Exercise Dependence Scale-21 (EDS-21) [3], which assessed her exercise addiction (EA) level. Her score was 100 (out of a maximum possible score of 126). The EDS-21 has three classification groups: (i) at risk for exercise dependence; (ii) nondependent and symptomatic; and (iii) non-dependent and asymptomatic [3]. Individuals who have scores of 5–6 on the Likert scale for at least three of the seven criteria (i.e., tolerance, withdrawal, intention effect, lack of control, time, reduction in other activities, and continuance) are at risk for exercise dependence [3], which Luna was experiencing. The therapist also sought information from Luna about her eating symptomatology based on the diagnostic criteria of DSM-5 [4]. Luna reported that her binge-eating behaviour did not occur on a regular basis, that it included certain types of food (e.g., sugary snacks), and that sometimes she could reduce the amount of food she ate. The therapist concluded that Luna's problems might represent 'unspecified feeding or eating disorder' [4]. Further examination with a group of questions based on the DSM criteria sought to exclude body dysmorphic disorder [4,5]. Luna reported no perceived defects or flaws in her appearance, although she tried to maintain her ideal body appearance.

It is important to highlight the differences between primary EA and secondary EA. In primary EA, the affected individual tries to avoid negative states, whereas in secondary EA the main purpose of physical activity is to regulate and manipulate body weight [6]. However, in reality there is not always a clear distinction between primary and secondary EA, because most people who exercise have concerns about their weight and body image [7]. Luna exercised continuously, independently of her eating behaviour.

Moreover, although one of the precipitating factors for exercising was to lose weight, the main perpetuating factor for her exercising behaviour was to deal with her negative emotions.

Since there is no consensus among researchers on the nature of EA and its place in the official psychiatric nomenclature, clinical recommendations for the treatment of EA have not yet been established [8]. However, cognitive–behavioural therapy (CBT) is the most commonly suggested treatment for EA [9], as it is for other addictive behaviours, such as gambling disorder [10] or internet addiction [11]. In addition, mindfulness-based relapse prevention practices have been found to be effective for both chemical and non-chemical addictions [12]. Therefore it was concluded that CBT techniques would enable Luna to understand how her thoughts, emotions, physical sensations, and behaviours interacted with each other, whereas mindfulness-based practices could increase her awareness of her 'autopilot' reactions to negative feelings, and help her to learn to tolerate those feelings. Mindfulness-based practices were incorporated throughout the 12-session course of online CBT treatment when necessary, as suggested by the literature [13].

12.3 Course of Treatment

After the initial assessment interview, the therapist focused on establishing rapport, briefly reviewing the results of the assessment process, discussing Luna's expectations regarding treatment, and identifying the goals of therapy in Session 1. Luna mentioned that she did not want to abstain from exercise altogether. The therapist helped her to identify the goal of therapy as doing exercise without compulsive feelings, and stopping herself when her binge-eating behaviour was triggered. The other focus of Session 1 involved the therapist exposing Luna to the CBT model and introducing the concept of automatic thoughts. The therapist then explained to Luna how to complete an automatic thought record sheet, and the importance of this.

In Session 2, the therapist and Luna worked together on her homework. Luna was not capable of distinguishing emotions from thoughts. She had a limited repertoire for labelling emotions, and did not notice the physiological aspects of these. For instance, she had difficulty in describing her physiological signs in situations in which she felt anxiety. Therefore the therapist gave her psychoeducation about emotions, including their nature and functions, as well as the differences in frequency and severity of emotions. Luna was asked to keep a record of her thoughts, emotions, behaviours, and physical sensations as well as the triggering events.

In Session 3, the therapist and Luna discussed the role of her binge-eating and excessive exercising behaviours. For example, Luna reported that one of her automatic thoughts just before going to the gym was 'If I don't work out today, I will feel bad and then I will eat unhealthy snacks all night. So, I have to do it'. The therapist helped Luna to realize that she engaged in the same behaviours when she felt certain emotions, such as anxiety, anger, and loneliness. Moreover, the therapist reframed those behaviours as emotional avoidance strategies that contributed to the problem itself, although they provided some short-term relief. Luna engaged in binge-eating behaviour after experiencing negative emotions, and then exercised excessively to deal with the subsequent feelings of failure. As the amount of exercise increased, she became concerned that she would risk feeling upset if she stopped.

In Session 4, the therapist showed Luna how to practise mindful emotional awareness, so that she could learn how to observe her emotions without judging them. After that, Luna and the therapist evaluated this experience and agreed how Luna could practise it between sessions. In addition, Sessions 4–6 focused on identifying and changing her distorted thinking through the use of a number of cognitive restructuring techniques. In particular, the therapist and Luna worked on the all-or-nothing and catastrophizing thinking styles that were contributing to her rigid exercise and eating behaviours. For example, she considered missing a workout to be a major failure, and she would be unable to pull herself together for the rest of the week. She also had positive attributions about doing exercise excessively.

In Session 7, Luna was very upset because she had sustained a leg injury during a workout, and would have to take a a long break from exercise. The technique known as *anchoring the present,* which refers to the practice of paying attention to what is going on around oneself in the present moment [14], was used as an in-session exercise to demonstrate how Luna experienced strong feelings about this situation. The therapist and Luna then discussed her patterns in the automatic appraisals. She was struggling with the idea that 'nothing means anything' because of her injured leg. Through the use of cognitive questioning, Luna came to realize that exercise had an underlying meaning of *success,* which was related to approval and love shown by others. The therapist gently encouraged Luna to test this belief on her interpersonal interactions in Sessions 8–10. Since Luna had to be withdrawn from workouts, this was an opportunity to test her beliefs about experiencing negative emotions when she stopped exercising. The therapist and Luna generated adaptive alternative appraisals (e.g., 'It is OK to feel upset sometimes') and coping strategies (e.g., phoning someone) to deal with her negative emotions.

In the last two sessions, the therapist and Luna evaluated the progress that Luna had made during treatment. Her scores were now 4 for the BDI (indicating minimal depression) and 11 for the BAI (indicating mild anxiety), and her EDS-21 score had decreased to 46 (out of a maximum possible score of 126). Luna reported that she was able to stop and say to herself 'I have a strong feeling, so what is going on now?', rather than engaging in an automatic response. 'Still, I have difficulty with some feelings and thoughts, but now I know that this is a part of life, and they will not stay with me forever', she commented. Notably, being able to perceive emotions as waves in the ocean with ups and downs made Luna's experiences seem more manageable.

12.4 Roadblocks in Therapy

Research has demonstrated an association between general perfectionism and problematic exercise behaviours [15]. Luna had a schema of unrelenting standards for herself and others, which led her to hesitate to try developing new skills. In this case, the core beliefs about having high standards were not targeted specifically, but in-depth work on this issue might have contributed to changes in underlying core beliefs. In addition, the people around Luna were also exercising excessively, so it was difficult to test her ideas about relying on appearance and set a new agenda, rather than working out. Moreover, she attended a session from the locker room of a gym. If the sessions had been conducted face to face, she would have had to prioritize her needs, which was one of our aims. Nevertheless, research has shown that online CBT and a brief mindfulness-based intervention are effective treatments [16,17].

References

1   Beck AT, Rush AJ, Shaw BF, Emery G. *Cognitive Therapy of Depression.* The Guilford Press, 1979.

2   Beck A, Epstein N, Brown G, Steer RA. An inventory for measuring clinical anxiety: psychometric properties. *J Consult Clin Psychol* 1988; 56: 893–7.

3   Hausenblas H, Downs DS. How much is too much? The development and validation of the Exercise Dependence Scale. *Psychol Health* 2002; 17: 387–404.

4   American Psychiatric Association. *Diagnostic and Statistical Manual of Mental Disorders,* 5th ed. American Psychiatric Association, 2013.

5   Wilhelm S, Phillips K, Steketee G. *Cognitive-Behavioral Therapy for Body Dysmorphic Disorder: A Treatment Manual.* The Guilford Press, 2013.

6   Egorov A, Szabo A. The exercise paradox: an interactional model for a clearer conceptualization of exercise addiction. *J Behav Addict* 2013; 2: 199–208.

7   Starcevic V, Khazaal Y. Relationships between behavioural addictions and psychiatric disorders: what is known and what is yet to be learned? *Front Psychiatry* 2017; 8: 53.

8   Berczik K, Griffiths MD, Szabó A et al. Exercise addiction. In: Rosenberg KP, Feder LC, eds. *Behavioral Addictions.* Academic Press, 2014: 317–42.

9   Petry N. *Behavioral Addictions: DSM-5® and Beyond.* Oxford University Press, 2015.

10 Gooding P, Tarrier N. A systematic review and meta-analysis of cognitive-behavioural interventions to reduce problem gambling: hedging our bets? *Behav Res Ther* 2009; 47: 592–607.

11 Young K. Treatment outcomes using CBT-IA with Internet-addicted patients. *J Behav Addict* 2013; 2: 209–15.

12 Witkiewitz K, Bowen S, Harrop E et al. Mindfulness-based treatment to prevent addictive behavior relapse: theoretical models and hypothesized mechanisms of change. *Subst Use Misuse* 2014; 49: 513–24.

13 Hayes S, Hofmann S. The third wave of cognitive behavioral therapy and the rise of process-based care. *World Psychiatry* 2017; 16: 245–46.

14 Barlow DH, Farchione TJ, Sauer-Zavala S et al. *Unified Protocol for Transdiagnostic Treatment of Emotional Disorders: Therapist Guide.* Oxford University Press, 2017.

15 Hagan AL, Hausenblas HA. The relationship between exercise dependence symptoms and perfectionism. *Am J Health Stud* 2003; 18: 133–7.

16 Ruwaard J, Lange A, Schrieken B, Dolan CV, Emmelkamp P. The effectiveness of online cognitive behavioral treatment in routine clinical practice. *PLoS ONE* 2012; 7: e40089.

17 Cavanagh K, Strauss C, Cicconi F et al. A randomised controlled trial of a brief online mindfulness-based intervention. *Behav Res Ther* 2013; 51: 573–8.

Chapter

The Story of My Life

Thomas Brosnan

13

About the Author

My name is Thomas Brosnan and I am a Behaviour Change Expert who specialises in Addiction and Relationships. For over 20 years now, I have worked extensively with individuals of all ages, couples, families and groups to help them uncover their truth, to take ownership of the present and connect to their future self. I have experience of working in both the public and private rehabilitation sectors, such as the NHS and the Priory and am also the founder of Thought Based Therapy.

I am extremely passionate about child welfare, personal development and mental wellness and firmly believe that if we don't have broken children, we are much less likely to have broken adults. As a result, I strive to implement, research and develop early intervention strategies for the benefit of all which is why I am proud to be part of this project and humbled to be able to contribute the following case study.

13.1 Introduction

Addiction, a word derived from the Latin term meaning 'enslaved to' is subjective and in general, complex to define. Therefore, the specific behavioural addiction that is known as exercise addiction (EA), which was first observed by Baekeland [1], has yet to be included as a mental disorder in either the *International Classification of Diseases* [2] or the *Diagnostic and Statistical Manual of Mental Disorders* [3] and as such, is worthy of classification as contended in this chapter.

Among the range of terms used, 'addiction' is considered appropriate by Goodman whose proposed definition suggests compulsion, preoccupation and restlessness [4]. Consistent with this, the author also subscribes to the components of addiction suggested by Brown and later by Griffiths where salience, tolerance, withdrawal, euphoria, conflict and relapse are relevant in equal measure. It is with reference to these variables that the subject's habits in this case study are analysed [5,6].

The work of Grant et al. has shown how behavioural addictions such as exercise, although controversial, are sometimes referred to as impulse control disorders – a class of psychiatric maladies characterized by impulsivity, an inability to resist temptation, a drive or an urge [7]. Consequently, according to Szabo and Griffiths, such tendencies highlight the distinction between healthy 'committed' and unhealthy 'risky' exercisers as individuals who are addicted to exercise engage in rituals which have detrimental effects on their lifestyle [8].

Unlike 'substance addictions', behavioural addictions involve no chemical compounds upon which a person becomes dependent. However, despite the absence of substances, the internal chemical effect, especially in relation to the brain's dopaminergic system is akin to the effects caused by drugs or alcohol [9]. Therefore, the impact on the addict can be just as pernicious as we shall see in the following case study.

In the UK, it has been widely observed through data collected by Leisure DB and research by Bouchard et al. that the 10.4 million people who have a gym membership consider exercise to be physically and psychologically bene-ficial to health [10,11]. Equally, Blaydon and Lindner report that up to 52% of triathletes flaunt this belief and work out to an extreme degree [12]. Here, the literature highlights the harm that excessive exercisers cause to themselves which leads researchers to conclude that exercise can be both harmful [13,14] and addictive [15].

13.2 Case Study

Samantha is a 36-year-old British woman and mother of two who is employed as assistant head and PE teacher at a primary school. Describing herself as an 'exercise addict', she favours running, high-intensity interval training (HIIT) and core exercise. Raised in a stable home, both of her parents worked in mental health care and she has a brother 6 years her junior. Currently 1.57 m in height, Samantha refuses to weigh herself as she feels that this would 'cripple' her emotional well-being. However, she asserts that her weight is 58.5 kg and her dress size is a UK size 8–10 yet emphasizes that she is usually a UK size 6–8.

Samantha describes herself as physically weak from a health perspective due to a hip injury she sustained while running in November 2019 and to an episode in August 2020 where she compromised her immune system and contracted meningitis, arguably by pushing her body to the point of exhaustion. She also comments that her body is 'wobbly', undefined and generally repulsive from an aesthetic perspective. This, appearing to reflect an inability to exercise because of the previously mentioned health problems as well as genuine feelings of disgust from an emotional viewpoint arising from said injury and illness and also, from the feedback from her son that 'Mummy has gone all squidgy'.

In terms of exercise, Samantha characterizes her behaviour as 'extreme' and describes having an 'all-or-nothing' attitude. There are times when she struggles with everything – her thoughts, her diet and her clothes. However, she comments that she would never 'let herself go' (e.g., by not training and thus gaining weight) which, implies a degree of self-control. At the other end of the extreme and prior to her hip injury, she pushed herself to the limit by striving to exceed her 'normal' 80 km weekly run, her five to six times a week HIIT sessions, and her four to five times a week core training sessions by squeezing in extra sessions where she could when she could. This, at the cost of declining or postponing social invitations by saying 'I have plans' when in fact, her intention was to train.

Having adopted a mantra of 'Eat less move more Eat more move more!', Samantha exercises hard to work off the calories she has consumed. She mentions her need to feel constitutionally proud of herself and strongly believes that everything could always be better in terms of her idea of body perfection. Observing her thoughts about being in control, the author hears her narrative about choosing to exercise for herself rather than it being an act that completely drains her. That said, the findings of Foster et al. [16] suggest that there is evidence of body dysmorphia in Samantha's discourse as she describes the physical pain she experiences as she insists her neck is too fat to the extent that she cannot wear a necklace because it would be too tight. She also states that walking is uncomfortable too as she believes her thighs are so large that she experiences 'chub rub'.

To highlight, Samantha's diet is strict and balanced and she is aware of the food-related behaviour that needs to be modelled for children. She sets good examples of moderation by drawing their attention to the rare occasions where mummy may have chocolate and explains that while nothing is off limits, it is important to be mindful of how much is consumed. That said, even though Samantha does not consider herself to have an eating disorder, it has been reported that up to 48% of people with EA exhibit disordered eating behaviours [17].

Commenting that her children are the most important part of her life, Samantha acknowledges that she has sacrificed her own well-being to exercise by ignoring medical advice to implement rest days when recovering from illness. However, whenever she ceased exercising for a nominal period of 2–3 weeks rather than following the prescribed advice that she should wait until she was 'fully recovered', her cognitive capacity was also affected as she experienced short-term memory loss. Samantha expressed her anger in the words life is getting in the way of being able to train' and it was at this point that the author respectfully enquired whether the children were as salient as she asserted given how she continually rationalized her behaviours in pursuit of perfection.

Samantha has a long-standing relationship with sports which stems back to the age of 6 years. From formal to further and higher education onwards, she has played football, netball and hockey. She also has a love for athletics and is a qualified referee, a football coach and a personal trainer.

During the conversation with Samantha, the author detected an overarching rebellious streak in her personality which underpinned her desire to prove people wrong that further demonstrated her determination. This, highlighting the steadfast attitude peppered throughout her life where she had defied the odds to overcome a broken collarbone in order to pursue a career in PE, battled chronic fatigue syndrome between the ages of 16-19, recover from a knee injury while studying for her GCSEs and, achieve a First-Class Honours degree when she was 21. All of which compounding the fact that when Samantha is told to do something like rest, she doesn't. Moreover, being 'told' not to do something or being told 'you can't is actually source of motivation for her and something which fuels her desire to do more or as Samantha would describe it, 'the story of my life'.

That said, in retrospect, Samantha reports having felt more in control when she was younger than she does now as she is constantly pushing herself to her physical limits to exercise while compromising the necessary periods for rest. For instance, she sets herself goals such as establishing a limit of doing 30-second intervals whilst listening to a song or giving herself a set distance to run or noting a time to get to a certain location. However, when these goals are reached, she continues. Thus, ignoring her own self-imposed limits and as we have seen, increasing the risk of injury. In spite of this cognitive dissonance, Samantha views such extensions of her goals as more of a choice than a compulsive behaviour. However, when challenged, she struggles not to exercise, even though she acknowledges the impulsivity of her own decision-making process.

Noting Samantha's metacognitive strategies (i.e., the information that she holds about her own internal state), the author concluded that her score on the Exercise Addiction Inventory [18], which was 24–30 (indicating a risk of EA), and her results on the Metacognitive Questionnaire [19], which showed that her two dominant metacognitions were cognitive self-consciousness ('I pay close attention to how my mind works') and beliefs about the need for control ('I need to control my thoughts at all times'), are consistent with previous research which has demonstrated that the need to control one's thoughts is a strong predictor of addictive behaviour [20]. Therefore, the author hypothesizes that metacognitions, particularly the beliefs that one has about the need to control one's thoughts may play a similar role in EA to that which they have in other addictive behaviours.

In addition, when faced with the prospect of not training, even for a day, Samantha feels that there is a significant negative impact on her mood and self-esteem and this leads to her avoiding social situations so that she will not have to wear certain clothes. Moreover, whenever it is impossible to avoid attending an event, she wears oversized garments to hide her body from public view. From a rational perspective, such behaviour only seeks to exacerbate her physical, psychological and/or interpersonal distress, consistent with the hypothesis proposed by Lichtenstein et al. [21].

This need for control is also supported by the endorphin hypothesis and the affect regulation hypothesis [22,23], as Samantha's attitude towards exercise leads to a positive mood state in which she 'trains to feel better' to alleviate her negative feelings relating to body dysmorphia. The theories proposed by Morgan and Schore are pertinent here [22,23], as they are consistent with the 'runner's high' phenomenon – the pleasant emotional state associated with positive self-image and the sense of control and fulfilment we observe in Samantha's narrative. This, leading to an increase in positive affect which contributes to her being more confident, assertive and seemingly grounded. All of which allowing space for her to process life – 'a clearing of the mind' as she calls it as this is her time to be her, to feel free, released and 'just me' rather than being Mrs X or a Mummy.

This, adding support to the author's hypothesis regarding Samantha's need to control her thoughts as she also experiences her highs in relation to her clothing too. For example, she feels confident when she looks great wearing T-shirts, vest tops and dresses that accentuate her figure, muscle tone and body definition. There is also the question of how she feels as a consequence of these harmful behaviours and the extremes to which she will go to in order to feel proud when the key question, 'Is it worth it?', is posed. Samantha maintains that it is, 'most definitely,' she replies as it is all about feeling accomplished and having strength of character which creates a powerful sense of self, but not egotistically she hastens to add as it is much more about how she feels within than it is about other people's perceptions. Hence the work of Donald Nathanson as he shows how emotions are triggered in private moments [24].

With regard to negative consequences and conflict associated with exercising, Samantha describes how her exercise fits in around her children and how it has affected them (e.g. how they struggled to cycle alongside her as she took them on runs during lockdown and how when abroad, they attended kids' club so that she did not have to miss a day of training). Samantha further shares how she would get up earlier and go to bed later in order to train which, had an impact on her ability to self-regulate as she would be deprived of essential sleep and this may have contributed to the cognitive impairment caused by the meningitis. She then admits that if her work still needed to be done, she would arrive home after her children had eaten which meant that family mealtimes were compromised too.

Samantha also describes how exercise caused hostility between herself and her former husband, to the point where they eventually separated. Memories of the experience of having meningitis led to thoughts about exercising. In continuing with the impact on her family, Samantha explains how exercise caused hostility between herself and her ex-husband to the point where they eventually separated after 14–15 years. This evoked memories of having meningitis she says which gave birth to thoughts of exercising sensibly that were soon dashed as despite the incessant urge to do more now that she could, she instead, came to the stark realization that her children now only had her.

However, this did not prevent her from exercising as the desire was obviously still there. However, it did deter her in terms of how long she would train for. Crucially, at this point Samantha mentions her fear that her children will one day wake up and find her lying unconscious on the floor.

Without referring to any specific 'relapse', Samantha recalls the significant times when she should have rested while recuperating yet did not do so and also recounts how she struggled to juggle training with teaching early in her career. She describes this as having been a complete 'fuck it' period – chasing a career, a marriage and ultimately, a body. However, all of this could not be achieved without sacrifices, and indeed there were; sleep, free time and, as mentioned, her marriage. Samantha describes having no guilt about this as she now had more time to exercise since her husband no longer needed to be considered. This was the ultimate justification for her that this is what she has to do – train!

Samantha now believes she has a very fulfilled life in which she is flourishing professionally and personally. She has a new relationship and acknowledges that the encouragement and support offered by her current partner are is helpful and that she is grateful for his feedback.

Warmly conveying how awakening this experience has been for her, Samantha reveals the extent to which her self-awareness has now increased to the point that the author feels that if she understands her own psychology this deeply and can actually see her own red flags, then she should be able to articulate to herself with ease, her awareness of being less in control than she thinks. That said, given what has been explored thus far, it is evident how contradictory yet resolute she is given the dissonance in her discourse.

Furthermore, Samantha recognizes that having meningitis has made her aware of the need to 'give herself a break and to not be so self-imposing'. Here, she appreciated that paying greater attention to the need to exercise to excessive amounts and having healthier strategies to bolster her confidence and self-esteem such as meaningful social interactions would support her overall mental health and would bring about some much needed balance to her life. Such approaches would be well complemented by a course of exercise reprogramming, motivational interviewing, and cognitive restructuring in the form of behavioural therapy to address the cognitive dissonance and body dysmorphic disorder. Collectively, these proposals would seek to incorporate the expectancy-based changes in an attempt to break the cycle of addictive behaviours presented by Samantha.

Although she has indicated that she is not sure whether this maturity will lead to any major change in her habits, Samantha is curious to find out whether she could train sensibly and how things may look in a few months' time. Moreover, still justifying her need to control, Samantha knows that this is the illusion of addiction and with that said, the author is hopeful that this work has helped her to see this whereby we can be optimistic that the story of her life from this day forward will be a much healthier one.

References

1　Baekeland F. Exercise deprivation: sleep and psychological reactions. *Arch Gen Psychiatry* 1970; 22: 365–9.

2　World Health Organization. *ICD-11 for Mortality and Morbidity Statistics*. World Health Organization, 2019.

3　American Psychiatric Association. *Diagnostic and Statistical Manual of Mental Disorders*, 5th ed. American Psychiatric Association, 2013.

4　Goodman A. Addiction: definition and implications. *Br J Addict* 1990; 85: 1403–8.

5　Brown RI. Some contributions of the study of gambling to the study of other addictions. In: Eadington WR, Cornelius JA, eds. *Gambling Behavior and Problem Gambling*. University of Nevada Press, 1993: 241–72.

6　Griffiths M. Exercise addiction: a case study. *Addict Res* 1997; 5:161–8.

7　Grant JE, Potenza MN, Weinstein A, Gorelick DA. Introduction to behavioral addictions. *Am J Drug Alcohol Abuse* 2010; 36: 233–41.

8　Szabo A, Griffiths MD. The Exercise Addiction Inventory: a new brief screening tool. *Addict Res Theory* 2004; 12: 489–99.

9　Fontes-Ribeiro CA, Marques E, Pereira FC, Silva AP, Macedo TRA. May exercise prevent addiction? *Curr Neuropharmacol* 2011; 9: 45–8.

10　Leisure DB. *State of the UK Fitness Industry Report*. Leisure DB, 2018. www .leisuredb.com/blogs/2018/5/16/2018-state-of-the-uk-fitness-industry-report-out-now

11　Bouchard CE, Shephard RJ, Stephens TE. *Physical Activity, Fitness, and Health: International Proceedings and Consensus Statement*. Human Kinetics Publishers, 1994.

12　Blaydon MJ, Lindner KJ. Eating disorders and exercise dependence in triathletes. *Eat Disord* 2002; 10: 49–60.

13　Deportivo EC. Perseverance and addiction processes: clues to identify exercise addicts. *J Concurr Disord* 2019; 1: 31–46.

14　Yates A. *Compulsive Exercise and the Eating Disorders: Toward an Integrated Theory of Activity*. Brunner/Mazel, 1991.

15　Szabo A. The impact of exercise deprivation on well-being of habitual exercisers. *Aust J Sci Med Sport* 1995; 27: 68–77.

16　Foster A, Shorter G, Griffiths M. Muscle dysmorphia: could it be classified as an addiction to body image? *J Behav Addict* 2015; 4: 1–5.

17　Hausenblas HA, Downs DS. How much is too much? The development and validation of the Exercise Dependence Scale. *Psychol Health* 2002; 17: 387–404.

18　Szabo A, Griffiths MD. The Exercise Addiction Inventory: a new brief screening tool. *Addict Res Theory* 2004; 12: 489–99.

19 Wells A, Cartwright-Hatton S. A short form of the metacognitions questionnaire: properties of the MCQ-30. *Behav Res Ther* 2004; 42: 385–96.

20 Spada MM, Caselli G, Nikčević AV, Wells A. Metacognition in addictive behaviors. *Addict Behav* 2015; 44: 9–15.

21 Lichtenstein MB, Hinze CJ, Emborg B, Thomsen F, Hemmingsen SD. Compulsive exercise: links, risks and challenges faced. *Psychol Res Behav Manag* 2017; 10: 85–95.

22 Morgan WP. Affective beneficence of vigorous physical activity. *Med Sci Sports Exerc* 1985; 17: 94–100.

23 Schore AN. *Affect Regulation and the Origin of the Self: The Neurobiology of Emotional Development.* Routledge, 2016.

24 Nathanson DL. *Shame and Pride: Affect, Sex, and the Birth of the Self.* W. W. Norton & Company, 1994.

Chapter

14

Money Honey
An Interview with an 'Informed' Patient
Silvia Rossato, Pierluigi Simonato,
and Angela Scoppettone

14.1 Introduction

This interview with a patient whom we shall call 'Money Honey' (or 'MH') was conducted in 2019 at our 'Parco dei Tigli' Clinic[1] in north-east Italy. The clinic can accommodate over 100 inpatients affected by psychiatric disorders (e.g., depression, bipolar disorder, personality disorders) and/or addictions (e.g., cocaine, gambling, novel psychoactive substances), and it offers specific and specialized programmes (e.g., psychopharmacological interventions, individual and group psychotherapy) for recovery from these diseases and disorders.

The Dual-Diagnosis Unit in which this case was assessed is dedicated to supporting recovery from both classic and novel substance and behavioural addictions, and revealing the psychopathology underlying the misuse of such compounds. In this case, alcohol use was comorbid with bipolar disorder and narcissistic personality disorder (assessed by psychiatrists and psychologists).

MH is a 32-year-old man who worked as a finance broker in Milan and then became the owner of several gyms, where he also worked as a personal trainer, giving 'information' to his clients on how they could best boost their physical performance by using a variety of products.

MH was admitted to our Dual-Diagnosis Unit twice, first in July 2014 (for 30 days of hospitalization) and then again in October 2019 for a shortened (10-day) programme. On both occasions he attended the Unit for stimulant and alcohol use disorder and an unspecified mood disorder. He had no previous psychiatric history. He described himself as having been a hyperactive child, and stated that he had been involved in several intense sports activities from childhood onward. He started playing football and basketball and was involved in karate and skiing at the age of 3 years. By the time he was 5 years old he was already involved in competitive sports (skiing and karate), and taking part in three workout sessions per week. He continued with these competitive activities, practising other sports (basketball, tennis, and football),

---

[1] www.parcotigli.it

and dedicating his summer holidays to intensive training, until he was 15 years old. He then gave up competitive karate and skiing, but he continued training in different sports (e.g., mixed martial arts). At the age of 29 years he started to attend a gym, engaging in three to four workouts per week, with each workout lasting for 1–2 hours.

During both hospitalizations the patient was assessed with the Addiction Severity Index (ASI), the Symptom Checklist-90-R (SCL-90) test/retest, the Beck Depression Inventory (BDI-II), the Structured Clinical Interview for DSM-5 (SCID-5-PD), the Alcohol Use Disorders Identification Test (AUDIT), the Exercise Addiction Inventory (EAI), and the Appearance Anxiety Inventory (AAI). Although the patient had a very intensive training routine (four or five times a week, for 1–2 hours), he did not have significantly high scores on the EAI and AAI [1,2].

The final diagnosis, according to the tests and clinical observation, was narcissistic personality disorder, stimulant and alcohol use disorder, and bipolar disorder not otherwise specified (BD-NOS).

14.2 The Interview

Therapist Good morning, MH. During the last interview we talked at length about your athletic activities and competitive experiences in skiing, tennis, and karate when you were a child. We then focused a bit more on your sports activities at the gym over the last 3 years. Can you confirm that you found out at the gym about the products that you use to enhance your workouts?

Money Honey Yeah sure, like I told you I started getting to know them through one of my friends, my right-hand man in the gym. He initially gave me proteins and glutamine, the basic stuff, you know, I was very focused on training and nutrition at that time. When I train seriously, I don't use cocaine, I'm very careful. I'm an all-or-nothing guy. If I get high, I just get high, I can't stop. However, if I decide to get in good shape, I just focus on that, and I'm really committed. At the beginning I lost a lot of pounds, I had a specific workout three times a week and then I would get my products, ordering them online. In addition to proteins, I started to enquire about taking something that would burn fat fast and allow me to perform at my best. At that point I put on muscle, see (he shows his arm), now I've lost everything, the last few months I messed up, but now I'm willing to get serious about this thing again. I can't see myself like this any more, I don't like myself at all and I miss doing physical activity, it used to give me an extra charge, working out gives me an insane boost.

T Yes, I understand. I realize that this all-or-nothing mode that you're talking about is something that we've referred to before, both in terms of relationships and work. So, when you were training, you started to enquire about how you could perform at your best, to learn about other products that could help you reach your goals as quickly and as well as possible. What are these fat-burning products? What are they all about?

MH We're talking about different types of products. Would you like me to explain?

T I'd like to understand more.

MH So, as I told you before, I was taking various types of *proteins* and *glutamine*, which combined are used for muscle building, and right from the start I felt that the training was giving more benefits, I was making progress quickly, combining a balanced diet. Then I started taking *clarinol tablets* before meals to burn fat (so in addition to putting on muscle I was sure to get rid of fat faster), *acetyl L-carnitine* before training or immediately after, that makes you give your best, especially in 'sprint' activities, and *creatine monohydrate* before high-intensity workouts. Then I used to take *phosphatidylserine capsules* to better boost my brain activity as well. The spearhead are *thermogenic products*, because those are really strong and act on the body, but especially on the mood, giving you a boost. Although those aren't exactly easy to handle and they cause irritability. I took them for a while and I felt really tense, like I was always ready to snap. Then it's a matter of experience, both for the thermogenics and for the others, you have to test them on yourself, try to see what works best for you as doses are indicative and create your own programme to take them. I jumped right in, when I set my mind on something, I pursue it to the fullest, there are no half measures, so I was experimenting, and I had good results too. I was just focused on that and I was really good at that time, things were going well for me, with the clients, with the girls, it was a really good time.

T I feel like you know a lot of things about these products. I had no idea there were so many alternatives. Were you managing any gyms at that time?

MH Yes, I started 3 years ago. I was running them with my friend, my right-hand man. I trained, I could choose which gym to go to and the more I trained the more satisfaction I got and I wanted to push harder. So, I learned all about products: the guys who were training at my gyms, whom I began training with, gave me good tips. Then I would do the rest, the gyms always have great contacts. I began researching and experimenting. In a year, I was able to give advice to clients on the best products to take and the new clients trusted me. I was able to find what I wanted. Milan is like that, it is all about image, and physical appearance is very important. So, if you can get the best in less time, it's a win-win. I was very clear with the guys on one thing, though: that you can't just take these products like that, unless you do serious training and follow a regular diet. You have to be careful about that, otherwise both the activity and the products are useless.

T It seems to me that you have a very clear picture. Certainly, over time you've expanded your knowledge and by trying different products you got a better idea of what works.

MH Of course, I used to keep track of things at the gym. I was advising the guys on what to take. It wasn't until a certain point that I realized that when it comes to thermogenic products you have to be careful. They're not easy to handle, especially for someone like me who doesn't stop, who doesn't quit until the very end. They started to give me some pretty big mood swings, actually even here at the clinic it got a little bit out of hand.

T You told me about it, what happened?

MH I went overboard. I started to feel particularly nervous, here at the clinic it didn't take much to make me explode: one wrong word and I couldn't handle the situation as well as I once could. I feel tension every day, but lately it seems to be getting worse.

T When did you stop taking the products? How come you changed your lifestyle?

MH I liked that lifestyle and it allowed me to perform at my best and feel cool. I felt very accomplished and had a lot of confidence, I didn't have a problem doing anything. I usually put on a good show, but I often feel ashamed. I get anxious when I relate to others because I feel like I always have to prove something. At that time though, I didn't feel the need to use cocaine to feel comfortable all the time, I was enough, I was always charged up. Then at a certain point I was even too loaded maybe. My friends would tell me that I never stopped and I wasn't that nice any more. I didn't have a brake. I felt like I was able to start having nights again, because girls would ask me out, crazy chicks from the gym, beautiful ones, I couldn't say no. So, when I went, I allowed myself to drink, to eat more than usual, and then I would go back to the gym to recover. I can't tell you exactly when I crossed the line, however, it did. The nights started getting longer and I started going to the gym less and less.

T Did you feel guilty about what was going on?

MH Yes, I felt like a jerk because I couldn't keep control of the situation, I had been slaving away so much and I couldn't allow myself to quit. So, I'd go back to the gym, I'd even take a little extra to pump up the muscle and recover, but then I'd go out again at night, drink a lot, and the next day I felt like crap again. I started feeling ashamed of myself again, feeling uncomfortable. To hold up more I started taking cocaine again, to be gorgeous, so they wouldn't see that I was drinking too much, that I was quitting. Then I'd go to nice restaurants, big clubs, where my clients were. I couldn't show up wasted.

T Was this the time when you started to lose control with substance use?

MH Yes, at that point I didn't control anything any more. I started the same cycle again, there wasn't a time when I didn't feel the need to drink and do drugs. I stopped with the gym, cut back on products. That was a really bad time. Again. Now though, I want to get myself back on track, I promise you.

T I understand, MH, that the lifestyle you had taken on during the gym period gave you satisfaction, but at the same time it led you to relapse. What do you think?

MH Maybe it did, maybe I pushed too hard, the problem is that I can't give myself a limit, there is no limit, ever. I have to do more. Whether it's with cocaine, whether it's with training, whether it's with products. Then it all falls apart.

T Could the irritability you mentioned earlier have also affected it?

MH It's likely. At the beginning I needed alcohol to ease my tension, to make me feel calmer. Then it escalated, because I've always had a problem with alcohol.

T OK, thank you. In the next meeting we will try to focus more on the relapse and the mechanisms that maintained it.

14.3 Final Considerations

During his recovery, MH described in detail the use of a variety of image- and performance-enhancing drugs (IPEDs) [1–3] by himself or by his clients in order to improve their performance [4], their appearance, and their image, especially during the gym sessions. He was considered an 'expert' on different compounds, and was able to suggest brands of products, ingredients, and a dietary plan, highlighting the 'balance' between fitness supplement purity and alimentation. He never used anabolic-androgenic steroids (AAS), considering them very dangerous.

MH provided a description of several products, as reported in the following list (in which he described the most reliable brands on the market):

1   Whey proteins: in powder form, 30 g for each administration. MH stated that they were 'useful for post-workout and suggested before sleep'.

2   Glutamine: powder form. 'Mix 2 scoops (5 g) with 200 ml of water or other beverages and take it once a day, during the day or after physical activity. Combine this integration with proteins but avoid consuming it in the evening'.

3   CLA (conjugated linoleic acid; Clarinol): capsules. '3 soft gels once a day with water. This supplement helps to burn fat and should be consumed before meals'.

4   BCAA (branched-chain amino acids: BCAA): leucine, isoleucine, and valine. 'Add 1½ scoops (5.5 g) in 150 ml of water or other beverages and take once a day before or immediately after workout or competition. On non-training days the product may be taken at any time of the day. You can consume these products five times a day; it helps build and regenerate muscles and also has a mental effect'.

5   [Brand name] (thermogenic product): in capsules, containing L-tyrosine, green tea (*Camellia sinensis*) leaves, cocoa (*Theobroma cacao* L.) seeds, theobromine, bitter orange (*Citrus aurantium* L. var. *amara*) immature fruit, synephrine, caffeine. 'Two capsules a day with water or other preferred beverage, preferably before meals or during the day. You get a strong effect using this product, particularly on your mood'. MH later disclosed that he had suspended the use of this product because of mood swings. He also experienced some physical (mainly gastrointestinal) side effects. He decided not to take it or to suggest it to his clients any more.

6   Acetyl L-carnitine: tablets: 'One tablet once a day with water or other beverages, before training or competitions or immediately after. I suggest a more intense use: one tablet in the morning, two pre-workout, and one in the evening. You will get a mild improvement, especially in the "sprint" activities'.

7   Phosphatidylserine (Phosphatidylserine Pro): capsules, one a day with water. 'The verified effect is an increased and overall better neuronal transmission at Central Nervous System level'.

8   Creatine monohydrate: powder form. '3.5 g at a time before workout; it has a good effect on repetitive, high-intensity, and short-duration activities'.

MH completed the entire (30-day) detoxification programme, with psychiatric and psychological interviews and both individual and group cognitive–

behavioural therapy for addiction. He was discharged with a treatment consisting of mood stabilizers and an intense aftercare programme.

This chaper has described the case of a patient who, as a personal trainer in his gyms, used several products himself and suggested them to others, providing information and tips on their consumption [1,2], even though he did not have any specific expertise in this field. It is important to emphasize that the different products or combinations of supplements were not used under medical supervision or medical recommendation.

MH had personality and mood disorders as well as addiction problems. He repeatedly admitted that the use of some products (especially thermogenic mixtures) affected his psychopathological state [5]. This suggests that the consumption of such compounds needs to be carefully evaluated and monitored in patients with psychopathological symptoms, especially those suffering from bipolar disorder [6].

References

1　Corazza O, Simonato P, Demetrovics Z et al. The emergence of Exercise Addiction, Body Dysmorphic Disorder, and other image-related psychopathological correlates in fitness settings: a cross sectional study. *PLoS ONE* 2019; 14: e0213060.

2　Dores AR, Carvalho IP, Burkauskas J et al. Exercise and use of enhancement drugs at the time of the COVID-19 pandemic: a multicultural study on coping strategies during self-isolation and related risks. *Front Psychiatry* 2021; 12: 648501.

3　McVeigh J, Evans-Brown M, Bellis MA. Human enhancement drugs and the pursuit of perfection. *Adicciones* 2012; 24: 185–90.

4　Rowe R, Berger I, Copeland J. "No pain, no gainz"? Performance and image-enhancing drugs, health effects and information seeking. *Drugs (Abingdon Engl)* 2016; 24: 400–8.

5　Schifano F, Orsolini L, Duccio Papanti G, Corkery JM. Novel psychoactive substances of interest for psychiatry. *World Psychiatry* 2015; 14: 15–26.

6　Strakowski SM, DelBello MP, Fleck DE, Arndt S. The impact of substance abuse on the course of bipolar disorder. *Biol Psychiatry* 2000; 48: 477–85.

Chapter

15

Bodybuilding Saved My Life

Andrea Corbett

When I was diagnosed with a mental health disorder in 2015, I never imagined that my life would change in so many different ways. The diagnosis caused me to be signed off work from my role as a secondary school teacher – a role that I had had since qualifying in 2005, that I loved so much, and that enabled me to educate and empower young people to be the best they could be not just in business and computing, but in their life as a whole. The day I resigned, my life was turned upside down. I do not remember much about the day the doctor confirmed my diagnosis and prescribed me antidepressants, but I do remember wondering how I was going to tell my family.

My pre-diagnosis life was going relatively well, or so I thought. I was a school teacher at an inner-London secondary school, and this was a career I thought I would never leave, as I enjoyed it so much. However, my home life was slightly unpredictable, especially living with my teenage son and being his sole provider. Life at home consisted of me taking him to football, and then running around trying to make sure my home was in order and my school work was complete. All of this was as close as I got to any form of physical activity. I never really gave physical activity or exercise any thought. I was not overweight (at the time my perception was that the gym was only for those who wanted to lose weight), and I never was part of a team or played any sports, even when I attended school. I used to have an excuse at every PE lesson as to why I could not take part, and I used to be the cheerleader for my friends when they competed in any form of sporting activity. I had no interest in getting sweaty for the fun of it. Walking was never on my agenda either – I would drive everywhere, even to the shops, although it would probably would have been quicker to walk by the time I had got the car ready and driven there.

As a result of my diagnosis, I had to make frequent visits to the doctor to report how I was feeling and to collect my monthly prescription for anti-depressants. On one occasion the doctor suggested that I should try going to the gym, as I was continually reporting no changes in how I was feeling post diagnosis. At first I was offended by his suggestion, as I thought he was hinting that I had a weight problem. This was quite possible in view of the amount of sugary food and alcohol I was consuming. However, it turned out that he was not referring to my physical appearance, but was suggesting exercise as a way to help to manage my mental (and overall) health. I pondered the idea for several days, but finally made up my mind when I thought about the benefits of restoring the mother–son relationship to what it had been before I was diagnosed. Effectively this was my 'Why'.

My first day in the gym was very strange, especially as I had become accustomed to not leaving the house (or even my bedroom). I did not stay for long, as it was a very strange environment. The next day I stayed longer, and this momentum increased daily as I started to feel that I was enjoying the gym – it gave me an 'endorphin rush' and a 'dopamine high'. I would sometimes visit the gym three times a day to get my 'fix'. It soon became the norm for me to attend the gym after getting up, going home to eat, and returning in the afternoon and then again in the evening. There were some nights, especially over the weekend (when I knew I did not have to get up early and attend to my son), when I would go in the middle of the night because I was suffering from insomnia and I thought it would be better to count reps than sheep. My family started to become worried about me, and often asked or made comments about me being addicted to the gym, or they would suggest that I was using the gym as a way to avoid dealing with my situation. My friends complained that I had started to spend more time in the gym than I did with them.

After a period of constantly spending time in leisure centres I decided that I needed 'more', I felt the need to try out more than just the basic machines. This was when I became a member of what some would call a weightlifters' gym. The majority of the people I was surrounded by were bodybuilding competitors. They were focused, rarely spoke to anyone during their work-outs, and were never short of workout ideas, whereas I had no idea what to do. I quickly built up the confidence to talk to the gym owner and make enquiries as to what these people were doing and why. I soon learned to understand the basic requirements for becoming a bodybuilder, or at least someone who wanted to step on stage.

Over time I made friends among many of the competitors, and we had numerous discussions about what I would have to do in order to compete in a show. First, I needed to train daily. This was not a problem, as my days lacked structure.

I set about learning as much about this sport as possible, I did my research, found a show in which I wanted to compete, and this became my goal. It gave me a valid reason for getting dressed in the morning, and helped me reconsider the foods and drinks I was consuming.

Family and friends could also see the changes, mainly the physical ones, and not everyone liked them. I was continually being told to 'tone it down' and was asked very hurtful questions, such as 'Why do you want to become so muscular?' and 'Do you want to be a man?' Many people laughed at me when I told them I was going to compete. I tried to ignore these questions and negative comments, but they did have an impact on my already fragile mental health. For a while I started to rethink my reasons for wanting to continue with this. My family and friends were brainwashing me into thinking I was making the wrong decision. Eventually I stopped attending the gym, in order to please those around me. As a result, I started to fall back into my old habits of binge eating and alcohol consumption. I decided to return to the gym after a few days, and now exercised even harder, thinking that I had to make up for the lost time. In fact I was probably worse than before. I was constantly thinking about the lost time and having panic attacks about the possibility that I had lost muscle due to taking time off. This caused me to practically live in the gym. Some would say I had an unhealthy relationship with the gym at this point, as nothing could keep me away. I would take my meals to the gym so that I did not have to leave. I was constantly weighing myself, and if it was off target I would be extremely angry with myself and work even harder. My anger started to cause problems at home, as I would take it out on my family, and at one point I was asked if I was taking drugs, because the situation was so bad. I shut myself off from my friends until they stopped contacting me, and eventually we drifted apart.

The day finally arrived for me to compete at the United Kingdom Bodybuilding and Fitness Federation (UKBFF) National Championships. This was the day that I got known for being a 'show-stopper', because halfway through my time on stage the judges paused and took what felt like forever to decide. Then, before I knew it, I was being escorted off the stage by the head judge. I had no idea what was happening, and all I could do was cry uncontrollably while trying to protest my innocence. I assumed they thought I had taken drugs, because my body was more muscular than those of the other women who had been competing for years. I thought I was being disqualified from the show, but in fact I was being moved to another category, as the judges deemed me too muscular for the category I had signed up for (Bodyfitness/Figure). Instead, they were suggesting that I should compete in the Women's Physique category. As a result of this switch, I won the competition and was crowned UKBFF Women's Physique Champion 2015. Winning this show enabled me to become the first woman in this category to represent the UK in the international amateur shows, with my first appearance taking place in Budapest in November 2015.

This new title gave me so much confidence in myself that I wanted to go back to training the next day, as I now had an opportunity to go further with bodybuilding. However, this came at a cost. The occasional comments became more frequent as my attendance at the gym increased, my diet changed dramatically, my lifestyle began to change, and the people I spent the majority of my time with were mostly bodybuilders. Those around me saw this change as something negative, and now that they had discovered I had been diagnosed with a mental health disorder they were beginning to question how I could have won the show with so little experience. I was constantly being asked whether I had taken any pharmaceutical supplements, and I was even asked if I 'juiced'. I naively said yes, and that person responded by saying 'I thought so'. When I questioned this response, they began to educate me about bodybuilding lingo. I had thought they were asking me whether I juice food, which is why I had said yes. This taught me to be less quick with my responses. I finally convinced this person that I did not 'juice' (i.e., take steroids), but soon the question became a regular topic of conversations, to the point that I had to upload the certificate I had received as proof of being a natural bodybuilder. I also had to inform people that the reason why I was being invited to the drug-tested competition was because I was a natural bodybuilder. Many people suggested that I should leave this federation and join one that specifically stated that it was exclusively for natural bodybuilders. I refused to be bullied into making the switch by other people. Although I managed to calm this conversation down, after a while I was soon up against the constant question 'Are you sure you're OK?' – the question people would ask when I told them I was going to the gym, especially if it was not for the first time that day. It came to my attention that a few people were openly suggesting that this was becoming an addiction, and that I could not stop myself from always wanting to be in the gym. At one point I started to second-guess myself to the point where I decreased the amount of time I spent in the gym, but I noticed that I was not as happy as before, and my 'gains' were also starting to decrease, or so I was telling myself. I now realize that I was conforming to what society was telling me I ought to be and do, when ultimately I should have continued to decide for myself. After taking some much needed time to look deeper into why I wanted to continue to train in the way that I was doing, I realized that to the outside world my behaviour could give the impression that I was becoming addicted to the gym and to this new lifestyle, whereas what was happening was that I was becoming an elite athlete and adopting the athlete's mindset. Such a mindset requires an athlete to make a full commitment to what they are doing, to be dedicated, to make sacrifices, and to consistently show up. When I began to take this mindset on board, positive things started to happen in my personal life, I was able to wean myself off the antidepressants, and I became the founder and director of Focus On Creating Your Ultimate Self CIC, which was set up to educate and empower communities about the benefits and importance of good physical and mental health. I wanted to have a way to give back to my community, while helping others to see that what I was doing was not hindering my life, but in fact enabling me to turn what was once adversity to my advantage.

Since winning the Nationals in 2015, I have gone on to reach top five in the European Championships in 2016 and 2017, and then in 2017 I was placed second in the UKBFF British Championships, which gave me the motivation to train even harder to become the 2018 UKBFF Women's Physique Champion, I was also awarded my Elite Pro Card. As a result, I was able to compete at the Arnold Classics in South Africa in my professional debut in May 2019. After this show, I decided to change categories and was fortunate enough to compete in my second debut in September 2019, but this time as a Figure competitor at the IFBB Elite Pro show in Greece.

Chapter

16

An Interview with James Hollingshead[1]

Exploring the Balance between Focus, Professionalism, and Addiction

Roisin Mooney

16.1 Introduction

I am a senior health psychology researcher and project manager, and for the last 8 years have also been a female fitness model. I have always sought solace in exercise, but discovered a passion for weightlifting 10 years ago. I began studying psychology in 2008, which fulfilled my critical mind and desire to better understand how people think and behave. In 2012, I graduated with a First-Class Honours degree and started working at the University of Hertfordshire. I continued work while studying for a PhD, which I completed in 2020. In September 2020 I started full-time research at the University of Oxford.

Over the last 10 years I have observed how the landscape concerning fitness has evolved, particularly with the rise of social media. A fine balance has emerged between harnessing the abundance of mental health benefits that can be gained from engaging in exercise and adopting a healthy diet, and attaining unhealthy extremes that may be positively reinforced in public domains but have grave consequences behind the scenes.

In addition, there is an overwhelming amount of information available about what it truly means to be healthy, accompanied by an underwhelming level of professional responsibility or accountability. There is little governance or clearly qualified, evidence-based support for those seeking a healthier lifestyle and, based on my observations, this can often lead to disordered eating, amenorrhoea, poor mental health, and extreme physical exercise.

I met James 'The Shed' Hollingshead in person whilst training in a different gym after a photoshoot. James is a huge inspiration, and well

---

[1] International Federation of BodyBuilders and Fitness (IFBB).

respected in the bodybuilding industry. In spite of the many challenges that 2020 presented – both personally and because of the pandemic – he has won not one, but two professional bodybuilding shows, in October and November 2020. In this chapter we discuss our thoughts about the fitness industry and the interplay between exercising (and more specifically bodybuilding), either for general health or as a profession, and mental health. We dedicate this chapter to Luke Sandoe, James's best friend and fellow professional body-builder, who tragically lost his life in May 2020.

16.2 The Interview

Roisin Mooney Tell me a bit about your relationship with a ? after bodybuilding.

James Hollingshead It was my way of being unique, when I started lifting there weren't many people doing that. I always wanted to be a professional athlete, and always had a desire to stand out, which sounds egotistical, but it's more of an awareness that you can be different. I didn't want to attract attention, I just wanted to live a life that no one was living. I want to be a unique bodybuilder. I want to bring something to the table that makes me different from my peers. I want people to come away from a conversation with me and think he is not the same as everyone else, and that's my drive. It's more of a personal thing that translates into the sport and other things. It's always been a well-being thing for me over everything else, the results, and how well you do in things are part of said well-being, if you're doing great in that area you will always do well.

RM How has your bodybuilding career progressed?

JH I competed every year for the last 12 years to qualify for the British finals. Whichever category I was in at the time I would try to go and win the finals. As early as 2009 I won my first British title, I was a junior (under 21) in Mr Britain. In 2014 I won my weight class in the British, and in 2017 I won my weight class and the overall title to earn my professional status in the IFBB. It took 9 years of constantly competing to get to where I wanted to get, it didn't happen overnight. I never focused too far ahead, I always just focused on that year. Nine years flew by because I was always preoccupied, I always had a goal, and the goal was to win. Imagine saying to someone 'You've got to do 9 years to get that certificate', they would be like 'Sod that!'. I feel like there is purity for bodybuilding that has disappeared because of social media. People want credit before they have done it, and I feel like a lot of people want instantaneous credit.

RM I agree, I think we live in a society that is perpetuated by a misguided pursuit of perfection, with a lack of appreciation or understanding for consistent work over a long time that precludes success. What did your life outside of bodybuilding look like when you first started?

JH Every job I did and every pound I earned went into bodybuilding. At 16 years old I was working, doing removals and crappy jobs, just to earn money to pay for chicken. Everything I cared about was just being able to put my efforts into being a better bodybuilder. The jobs never meant much to me, they were always just a means to an end, to pay for bodybuilding. I never had any career in mind, I never chased a job and thought that would be my job, I chased bodybuilding. There was never a time when I changed that mindset. It has taken me 12 to 13 years to be able to earn money from bodybuilding, it's finally now actually given me a life. It's weird thinking back to those times because I almost can't remember them, it's like a life I never had, everything was for bodybuilding, it was all or nothing. That's why I love bodybuilding as I think of everything that it has given me.

RM That must have been challenging at times. How do you think you have maintained or developed your mindset throughout your career?

JH Just pride. I'm always the kind of person to evaluate how far I've come, and I would get annoyed at myself if I knew there was more in the tank. It's knowing that I have more to give, and I would never accept stopping short. I know in bodybuilding, to be a winner isn't just about being the best, it's about being the person that can endure. There will be many people in sport that are better than you, but if they don't have the mindset, and they give up, they disappear and then there is a gap, and you can fill that gap. You have to believe in yourself. If you truly have something in your gut telling you that that's the right thing to do, that means more than anything, that means more than your parents' words, that means more than your best friends' words, because even those people sometimes have doubt.

RM I think whilst other people may influence you, ultimately you are responsible for your choices and actions. You have to be accountable to yourself to ensure that how you behave aligns with your goals. Where do you think that we can draw the line between exercising for well-being, or a job, and an addiction?

JH Time. People spend hours exercising, people go to the gym more than once a day as a release, and without realizing that it isn't their release, it's their shackle. I see that a lot with females. I've seen a lot of females get really fit and then it goes beyond that, and they are so addicted to being light and trim and thin. Then you get the males who rack up massive debts spending copious amounts of money on pharmaceuticals and being obsessed with grow, grow, grow. I think that it is very easy to fall into that place if you are someone who hasn't been educated on the importance of balance. The problem is that a lot of people are educated to the point where they think that more will result in or lead to better results. It gets to a point where they feel guilty, they tell themselves 'I can do more, I should do more'. I've been there, I used to do cardiovascular exercise two to three times a day when I was preparing for shows on top of weight training, and I would spend the majority of my time in the gym. My mindset was the more I give to this the more it's going to give back, but that's not the reality. The reality is smart planning and knowing when to push and when to pull. So I think there is a real issue in terms of educating people about balance.

RM I think social media can be a real catch-22 with education. There are a lot of people putting out really good content who are well qualified and very talented in applying that knowledge in a way that people can access. However, there is such an overwhelming amount of content that people have access to, you have to be motivated to find it. On the other hand, I think that social media can be a real driver for exercise addiction, you see the highlights and you don't always see the hard work and resilience behind that.

JH That's the frightening thing. I know young individuals that want to be bodybuilders, who started training this year and you ask them 'What do you want to achieve next year?', and they say 'I want to be a pro'. For some reason, everything in between has been dissipated. Everything is results, two pictures next to each other, and that is all people see. There is a lack of quality content explaining the interim, and I think the more that people explain that things take time, then maybe we would have more of a patient environment. When I used to watch bodybuilding VHS videos, they would show you the bodybuilder at the beginning of the diet and at the end. You would never know what happened in between, they never told you how many meals the person has to eat, how many hours of cardio, or how long it's going to take. It goes back to someone who goes to the gym three to four times a day because they think that more is going to make it happen quicker. It's the same with drugs – more drugs make it happen quicker. It's not necessarily stupidity, although the information is out there, it's clouded amongst other content, and it's hard to pinpoint. If someone on social media has an excessive following, what they say becomes fact. If enough people say that this is the way, it becomes the way. When someone has a million followers because they're pretty or because they have got a good physique, when they say something it becomes like a bible, and that is an issue. You have to be very aware that it is going to take a while, because if you search the fast way you will find the fast way. That way unfortunately is always the way that is going to cause the most damage to the human.

RM I think people's perception of time and their goals is really important. What protective factors do you think there are for people with a good mindset around exercise, people who enjoy exercise regularly and don't become addicted?

JH I always wonder about the ability to not allow things to become addictive or destroy you or be negative. Is that a trait that is in your genes, or is that something that has been nurtured through your experience in life? We are talking about all these people and their fitness lifestyle and how it makes them feel, but then we also have to consider their life. Outside of that, what has caused them to be in the position that they are in? Someone might be addicted to the gym because he had a tragedy earlier in his life and it was the one thing that made him feel like he could cope, another person might have had no tragedies, but they just get a buzz from overdoing everything, so it could be two totally different reasons but the same end result.

RM Everyone has a unique experience, but I guess we need to consider the commonalities in those experiences. From your observations of the fitness industry, what do you think the key indicators of exercise addiction may be?

JH I think if you have the choice of socializing with loved ones or the gym, and it gets to the point that you never socialize because you would rather go to the gym. I've seen that a lot, I've been there a little bit in the past, but the only time I've been there is when I'm prepping for a show that is going to boost my career. It's kind of weighing up should I see these people today or should I do the tasks that are potentially going to make my career move forwards, that's where it becomes difficult on a professional level. Luke used to feel a lot of stress, he earned good money, but he always had a fear of what will happen the day this stops. I can imagine that pressure to perform and to bring results can sometimes be overwhelming.

RM Do you think professional bodybuilders could be addicted to exercise to the extent that it would have a detrimental impact on the rest of their life?

JH Definitely, I would say that they are the ones you probably don't see much of because it has taken away their ability to present themselves in a good light, so you won't see them because they are struggling. The mainstream bodybuilders, the ones that you see on Instagram or just in general, are the ones that are doing the best job of balance. There are many, many, many dark stories of bodybuilders. It happens to many before they even become professionals, like people that are on their way up. It is all or nothing because of everything it involves. Some people go beyond the extremities, and when those extremities are pushed there are so many implications, and those can be from health to social, mind, paranoia, anxiety, and body dysmorphia. Anyone that has pushed it too hard will have those things floating in their head and they will be in a dark place, you won't even know about it because they can't communicate with people. It happens a lot, and then the addiction to training itself. These people are very addicted to pushing their limits and getting in the gym and do stuff, a lot of them are broken because of it, because of overdoing everything. It is very prevalent. The number of people who have ended their career when they could have been something great, just because they have overdone it. Luke, bless him, earlier in the year had to lift a bit too heavy and tore his pec. He made a mistake on one exercise, on one day, and went a bit too heavy. Some people will do that day in and day out, and put their body through too much on a daily basis. The only thing about being a professional is I suppose there is you're getting paid, so you feel like you owe it to yourself to push to such extremities because there is financial gain.

RM So, I think the key message overall is that anyone is susceptible to exercise addiction. There needs to be more education surrounding balance and improving the understanding of what achieving professional status as a bodybuilder and maintaining a healthy mindset truly entails.

Section 3

Chapter

17

An Interview with Dave Crosland[1]
A LIfe with Performance-Enhancing Drugs
Valeria Catalani

17.1 Introduction

I had the pleasure of interviewing Dave Crosland ('The Freak'), a 49-year-old British professional bodybuilder who is currently actively involved in performance-enhancing drugs (PEDs) harm reduction in the bodybuilding community. Recently he turned his years of experience and usage of PEDs into an online professional service to help people. His goal is not to stop people using PEDs, but to educate them about responsible consumption and usage. In fact, he strongly believes that knowledge will reduce the harm and severe side effects caused by using PEDs. As he states in the following interview, he does not think that bodybuilding or indeed other sports disciplines can ever be separated from performance-enhancing practices. PEDs are what make professional sport sensational: 'If you take drugs out of the sport, there will be no sport'.

17.2 The Interview

Valeria Catalani When did you first become involved with the sport and fitness world? Was it through bodybuilding/weightlifting or through other sports disciplines?

Dave Croslands When I was 16 [in 1987] I started playing rugby for the school team. My brother had a set of weights in the cellar of our house, so I started using them, initially to supplement playing rugby. I was not a particularly strong person, even though I was a big lad, so my goal was to increase my strength for rugby. But then I realized that I enjoyed weightlifting – the challenge, and the training that went with it. Moreover, I was good, really good at it, and it soon became my focus because I was never particularly good at sports.

---

[1] Founder of Croslands Harm Reduction Services, http://croslands.org.uk/, in the UK.

VC Did you always want to become a bodybuilder, and where did this desire come from?

DC I always admired those cartoon physiques of He-Man and the like, but I didn't consciously decide to become a bodybuilder. Indeed, growing up, I was influenced by the positive superhero stereotype of masculinity – strong, muscularly lean, athletic, and body-perfect physiques – but my motivation was the training. I realized how much I loved it, and therefore I started my journey in this discipline. Of course, very soon in this journey, I started admiring bodybuilders' bodies. I always believed I could get very very big.

VC What were your ambitions when you started, and were your family, school teachers, and peers supportive?

DC When I got into bodybuilding, I was determined to turn professional and earn a lot of money from it. My opinion on bodybuilding is that it is a personal pursuit of discipline and you do not need family or friends' support for it. In a way it pushes you away from them. When I first started at 16 my parents thought it was just a phase and they tolerated it [diet and training], but they never encouraged me. My mum often complained about my eating habits, but on the other hand she helped a lot supporting my training. You could definitely say they were not supportive, but not against it either. However, when I started getting serious about my training I was no longer living at home, so there was no real family conflict.

VC Were your parents ever worried about you and your health, when you were getting involved in a sport that is often linked to the use of performance enhancers?

DC No, they weren't, they were ignorant about the subject and never considered that I could be using steroids. I was only 152 kg at that time, so it never entered their thoughts. They simply did not know.

VC When did you first become aware of performance enhancement in bodybuilding?

DC I started becoming aware of steroid use in bodybuilding when I was 16 or 17 years old, very soon after I started training. I was working out in a gym that, even if local, had a lot of high-calibre pro-level bodybuilders training there. I was spending 16 hours a day there and I was privy to a lot of conversations. They were never technical, in-depth ones, but were about what people were on.

VC Did those conversations include information about dosages and frequency?

DC The conversations were mostly general and private. They discussed what they were on and the amount, but not what it did or how it worked. Even though I was training with high-calibre bodybuilders who made me aware of doping, at that time I didn't know anything about the drugs, only that people were using them. No discussion was particularly on with peers, more with older and more experienced bodybuilders.

VC Can you explain the events that led you to begin to use anabolic steroids?

DC When I first started training, I didn't use any steroids. At that time, naive as it sounds, I genuinely believed that the difference between me and a professional bodybuilder was the training. Of course, as discussed before, I knew steroids existed, but I did not know back then how massive their impact on performance can be. So at that time I just motivated myself to train harder. I was really lucky to have the chance to train with very experienced bodybuilders. I learned a lot about how to train, and when you train with guys that are 'God', the training is extremely intensive. I had the so-called 'baptism of fire' with those guys, and everything was reaffirmed that it was all about training and training and training. Drugs were not the key element. This created for me a massive mental and physical foundation, a work ethic that was second to none. I started competing, and won the British title as a junior. However, after that, no matter how hard I trained, I did not feel there was anywhere left to go, so I decided to start using steroids. That was mainly because of my inspiration to go pro, and the decision to use was because I knew it would allow me to train harder. My passion was training. I wanted to push myself further, and I knew I couldn't do it without the drugs.

VC What was your mental process regarding this decision? Did you feel any pressure from your peers to engage in doping?

DC I am not sure there really was a mental process. I just wanted to be able to train harder, and using steroids would have enabled that. That was it, I did not give it much thought. There were not any other influential factors [home life, private life, school life] at the time. I did not feel any pressure back then from my peers, both when I felt I wanted to stay clean and when instead I decided to start to dope myself. Thinking about it now, I was probably influenced by a guy called Kev Taylor, three times British champion. That guy was an experimenter, and I was probably one of his experiments. However, during the time I was using, I was mostly deciding what to buy and what to use.

VC Was body image a motivator in your use of performance- enhancing drugs, or was it predominantly performance influenced? Do you think body image is an influential factor for bodybuilders?

DC At that stage, my motivation for using steroids was only performance based. So initially I did not have any real concern about my image, but as I progressed and developed, appearance became way more important. I was buying magazines and admiring those pro athletes, and yes, I used them as an inspiration and motivation for my training, but it was never just about body image. All bodybuilders are concerned about image, it is the basic driver of why they bodybuild. There is a difference, however, between competitive and non-competitive bodybuilding. For the latter, body image is the main driving factor. For competitive athletes, body image plays a role as well but it is more about trying to create a physique that is ideal. They are indeed image-conscious, but more around the parameter they need to look at their best for their competition. Non-competitive athletes instead are driven only by ideals, images that however are vague and very personal.

If body image is not a reason to start it, then it definitely becomes a factor when you get into bodybuilding. People are bombarded with pictures, comparisons, and lots of before/after posts, and start to get more and more self-conscious and critical. The relatively balanced image issues [a healthy and natural desire to change] that these people had at the beginning inevitably got turned into serious issues with a slightly obsessive edge.

Moreover, today's bodybuilding environment is very different from the one in which I grew up. Bodybuilders do not care about training or dieting anymore, they are not prone anymore to hard training and sacrifice. They only care about their image and how using steroids will help them achieve that.

VC Was anyone aware of your decision to use performance-enhancing drugs? Were you concerned about the potential ethical implications?

DC Some of my gym friends were aware of my decision. However, no one judged me negatively for it. Back then the bodybuilding environment was very good, everyone was supporting and helping and ready to cheer others' victories and achievements. I had no concerns about ethics, as there were no ethics involved. I was not claiming to be natural, and I wasn't going to try and compete as a natural. Generally, there are no ethics involved in steroid consumption in bodybuilding because it is just an accepted part of this discipline. We have tested federations for clean athletes and untested federations for the ones who use doping. There is no stigma attached to doping in untested federations. However, there is always someone who is cheating, and trying to compete in the tested federation even if they are using. I don't agree with this conduct and I think it is unfair. If there are rules, rules need to be followed.

VC Did you receive any advice about the potential health risks associated with usage before you started?

DC Back then there was no perception among my peers of how dangerous these substances could be. No one was talking about side effects or the negative impact of their usage, so I didn't think about it at all. There was no advice available from medical professionals or online. To be honest, even now medical professionals generally don't have a clue about steroids' side effects, and tend to come out with sensationalistic rubbish due to their own very poor knowledge. When I first started, I had no idea about steroids, shutdown, the impact on the endocrine system, or anything about the health risks associated with their consumption. I didn't know there were any health risks at all. So I had no concerns about steroids, and I didn't discuss the subject with anyone. I think I was just very lucky back then because I got access to very good-quality stuff.

VC Which substances were you using?

DC I had no idea. I did not use much but I had no idea what I was using. It was just a case of going to 'the guy' and asking what he had that was good, and that was what I used. I started my first cycle at 19 and finished it when I was 24. During those years I was running two injectables, changing them every 4 weeks or 6 weeks, with no understanding of the mechanism or side effects. I was taking something for 6 weeks, and if it worked and made me bigger, good. Otherwise after the 6 weeks I just changed it for something else. I was running on dosages of 1 gram for 4 years. In the end I was a monster, strong, relatively fit, and I looked pretty good.

VC How often were you training? Did you ever feel addicted to your training?

DC When I trained, I worked a three-on-one cycle. This means I was training for 3 days consecutively and then had a day off. I was doing only one session a day, and usually a session would last between 2 and 2½ hours. I was quite religious about this schedule, and I didn't like to miss any of my training. You can say I was addicted to it, but I enjoyed it, so it was never a negative addiction. I always went to great lengths to make sure I didn't miss scheduled workouts, even to the point that

I didn't like changing training times. I used to get really irritated if it happened, but that was because I wanted to progress and obviously a missed workout was a wasted one. I never used exercise to calm my nerves on purpose, but training was my stress relief. I have always been a very aggressive trainer, and I have always pushed very hard. That became very therapeutic. I never went to the gym thinking about problems, but I always battered myself to the ground and after that I would always come out extremely relaxed and chilled out.

VC Why did you stop then?

DC I injured myself, with complete detachment of the left pectoral muscle. The doctor decided not to reattach it because he could tell I was on steroids, and my career was over.

VC Do you think you injured yourself because your muscles were too big due to the steroid usage?

DC No, I don't think that I injured myself because of that. My pectoral was already damaged, but it was a moment in my career when I finally had the opportunity to become a pro. So I got back to the gym even though not feeling 100% and pushed as hard as I could, and my pectoral detached. I then came off everything. I didn't do any PCT [post cycle therapy], nothing. I just came off.

   It was not easy for me to stop training because that meant my career was over. After stopping using, I found myself left with very low levels of testosterone, depressed, and run down. I gained a lot of fat as well, but I didn't know what was causing all these effects. My personal life was an utter mess, and I got myself into a lot of problems. I didn't think it was particularly due to the steroids, but they were not helping because they were causing the low levels of testosterone.

VC What caused you to return to performance-enhancing drugs more than 10 years after quitting? Were you still practising bodybuilding during that period?

DC I got back into training after 13 years because I went to prison for VAT evasion. When I got to prison my life was a mess, I was fat and unfit, and I decided that the first step to pull myself together was to start training again. I stayed clean for 3 years. Then I opened a gym, invited some old friends who were professional and competing at that time, and they pushed me towards competing again. I knew that if I wanted to push myself further, I needed to start using again and that is what happened. This time, however, I started to document myself. Those were different times when people were talking more about steroids, and that made me realize that I wanted to know more about them myself. It was then that I started my journey towards my current job in harm reduction.

During my training to become a pro again, I realized that I didn't have enough motivation and that what I wanted was something else. I wanted to see how big I could get. I decided to film two documentaries to record my transition. I was determined to take as many substances as I could. To be honest I thought I was going to die. In my first documentary, I started with 1 g of testosterone and 500 mg of Deca and peaked at 3 g of testosterone and 1.5 g of Deca, reaching 165 kg. However, I still believed I could get bigger than that. I was already a 'monster', but the goal was to transition to 'freak'. I started a new cycle with 3 g of testosterone, swapping the 1.5 g of Deca for 1.5 g of trenbolone and using 27 IU of pharma-grade growth hormone and 120 IU of insulin per day. With these I managed to reach 188 kg. I had never taken so many drugs before, in my head was all or nothing.

VC Have you experienced any particular health problems related to usage?

DC I have, and it is the reason why I had to stop steroids for the second time. I had heart failure and stage 4 kidney failure, both because of my usage. However, the heart failure was potentially avoidable if I had not just stopped training. The kidney failure happened while I was filming my second documentary. My only goal back then was to get as big as I could. At that time, I experienced for the first time what is called the 'drug focus'. I was not relying on diet or training anymore. I was 165 kg and the only thing I was thinking about was what else I could possibly use or take to get even bigger. I wasn't thinking about anything else, I wasn't scared for my health, I just wanted more drugs to get massive. Then when I reached 188 kg, my kidneys failed. I stopped using immediately after that, but I continued to exercise. When I decided to stop exercising as well, being tired of going around at such a big size, was when I got heart failure. My heart was not fit anymore to pump blood in such a big body. I think that if I had kept fit, I would definitely have avoided heart failure, as it is not strictly connected with doping.

VC Have you observed or been made aware of other bodybuilders who suffered heath problems due to consumption of performance-enhancing drugs ?

DC Yes. All I deal with are users who have messed themselves up. That is pretty much what my job is – a harm reduction service. If someone messes themselves up with steroids they come and see me. Right now, the biggest growing area of health impact is the kidneys. I am regularly seeing users with significantly reduced eGFR [estimated glomerular filtration rate], acne, water retention, headaches, high blood pressure, and hypercoagulability. Steroids are tricky. They do not immediately cause health problems, they gradually develop them. In the beginning, you start with very mild side effects – water retention, headaches, acne, and high blood pressure. Your blood pressure can rise when you are on a cycle. It is not particularly worrisome if it is not persistent. However, if it is, it can cause severe damage to the kidneys. The same goes for blood – it thickens with anabolic steroid usage, increasing the chances of stroke. However, the side effects for most people who use are just inconveniences. Most importantly, users tend to overlook some common simple side effects, thinking that they are normal because they are on steroids. It is when they are left unchecked for too long that they can cause serious health problems. You have another area though that is particularly important and needs to be mentioned – mental health. Steroids have a very bad impact on the brain. From the nandrolone family, for example, Deca reduces the number of neuropeptides, impacting memory transference. Older guys who were doing the classic testosterone–Deca cycle now have a very serious memory issue. Trenbolone, probably the most famous steroid, is very powerful and very toxic, causing a high level of anxiety, insomnia, and very aggressive outbursts. It is directly toxic to the kidney as well, something I experience often with people who use trenbolone. Extended anxiety after stopping trenbolone, which has been shown to cause brain damage such as Alzheimer's disease, has been reported as well by users.

VC What is your perception of the health risks associated with performance-enhancing drugs? How do you explain the perceived absence of risk consideration related to the use of these substances in the bodybuilding environment?

DC There is a wide range of risks, as I mentioned before, but I think the risks are even more than the ones we know. We do not have an example of side effects linked to the use of steroids for different reasons. In the past, there has always been a taboo about openly admitting the use of anabolic steroids in hospitals or to doctors. Patients will not admit their usage to medical professionals due to a fear of prejudice, a fear that is well founded, too. Now, instead, people who use steroids do not even look as if they are using anymore, so when they present any side effects no one will think these are connected to steroid doping. I believe that we have yet to learn whether steroids can be used, and if the risks can be successfully managed.

However, to manage risks, we have to be aware of them, and many are not, particularly with regard to the impact that anabolic steroids have on mental health.

The absence of risk is a complex topic. To be frank, a lot of people are just dumb, but then you have a lot of disinformation on social media as well. I personally think no one is intentionally trying to mislead people. There is just not enough knowledge around. We have influencers saying that there are very few risks, and influencers who are trying to document themselves in order to share better information on steroids. As I said before, I think this is because people do not like to admit their usage, which results in an inaccurate risk assessment.

VC Do you personally have any health concerns for the future?

DC I don't have any particular concerns for the future. I took risks and I pushed the limits of what was physically possible. I knew I was not going to come out of that without damage. To be honest I am surprised I'm still alive.

VC Did your perceptions about steroids change over the years? What are those perceptions now?

DC Yes, they totally did. When I first started, I knew nothing about anabolic steroids, their mechanism of action, and their side effects. But when I came back after almost 13 years, as I educated myself, I became more aware of the risks associated with their usage. Even then I still had an 'It won't happen to me' kind of attitude. Now I know that these compounds demand respect and they can cause serious health problems. However, I never changed my mind about the fact that their responsible usage is mandatory for attaining levels of fitness and training that are out of reach for natural athletes.

VC What would your advice be now for individuals who are considering using performance-enhancing substances?

DC I am not against nor am I pro using them. If someone wants to use them, they should educate themselves and make informed decisions. I have seen very positive stories of people using anabolic steroids to improve their confidence in sports, and this resulting in improvement in their work and personal life as well. But I have seen very bad stories, too, with teenagers compromising their kidneys or their heart due to incorrect and irresponsible usage. I totally understand why someone who has dedicated their entire life to being the best in their discipline would consider using drugs. Taking some pills that will help you to achieve that goal for which you have been working so hard is a temptation too hard to resist. I personally think that elite athletes across various disciplines are currently using performance-enhancing drugs, and that federations are aware of it. I would not condemn this practice if it is done with a harm reduction approach. Ultimately you cannot stop people using them.

VC In your opinion, are there any ways in which these substances could be better regulated in bodybuilding, and in sports in general?

DC The use of steroids in bodybuilding is well regulated because the industry tends to regulate itself. When we see severe health problems, in general these are in people who are not athletes, but casual users or body-image users. Across the broader spectrum of sports, I am not sure. There was a proposal to allow doping in some disciplines, with usage limited to within certain ranges. However, I am concerned that if we allowed the open use of steroids, we might not see any difference in performance. How can we be sure that elite athletes are not already using a regulated form of doping?

Anyway, I think the first step towards better regulation is education. I think education needs to start in schools, but it needs to be honest. Our aim should not be to scare, but to inform. I have given several interviews for various organization, from Sky to the *Guardian* and more recently for Myprotein, and they are nearly always edited so as to paint steroids in a completely negative light. This does not educate – it just turns people away from support because they lose faith and trust in that information stream. I think it is pathetic that organizations do not have the courage to be honest and open about the use of performance enhancers.

VC Assuming everybody would agree, could you envisage a performance-enhancer-free environment for bodybuilders in the future, or is this inherently not a consideration due to the 'bigger is better' nature of this discipline?

DC Why would bodybuilding ever need to be steroid-free? As I said before, we have tested and untested federations, and you compete in them according to whether you are using or not using. The big bodybuilding shows (e.g., Mr Olympia) are untested, to keep them sensational. People want to see amazing performances. No one wants to see pro athletes who are just a bit better than average. If you get rid of enhancers in sports, sports will get boring.

VC And to conclude, do you regret using performance enhancers?

DC No, because it brought me to where I am now. I do not regret what I have done, or the drugs I have taken, because I quite like where I am now. I enjoy my job – it is a positive one, I do good, and I help people. Of course it is financially rewarding, but it is emotionally and morally rewarding, too. And let me tell you, you do not get that enough these days. It is worth it. If my journey had not been what it was, I would not be here.

Chapter

Being Comfortable in Your Own Skin
18
Oluyinka Idowu

It wasn't until I was asked to write this chapter that I truly reflected and realized just how much my life as an elite performing athlete contributed to my body self-image and mental health. Very early on in my life I was propelled into the world of elite sports.

I will start by giving a little background to set the scene, but what I will go on to explain will demonstrate how cruel and nasty the world of elite sports and people can be, and just how it affected my confidence, self-image, and general mental health.

I have never been what you would call a slim person. My body shape is curvy, and I have very strong thighs and musculature. I was what you would call a power athlete. At my best, I could squat 100 kg and bench 60 kg, holding my own with any male athlete my age. I was not that focused on my athletics, so I ate what I wanted, did not go to training if it was too cold, raining, or snowing, and besides I was at boarding school and had my homework to do. So long as I kept winning, I felt that my formula worked so there was no need to change.

I was what was considered a junior protégé and star. I became the British number two long jumper at 16 years of age, jumping 6.6 m by chance at some random event for my club. I don't know how I did it, and sometimes I was not that consistent in jumping big numbers because I simply did it out of sheer talent and nothing else. Suddenly all eyes were on me. I won the Junior Athlete of the Year Award, which I collected from Prince Philip at Buckingham Palace. I was regularly in the media doing well. I simply couldn't lose to anyone my age or even to most senior people, not because I was a dedicated athlete who worked extremely hard, but because I was very talented. I don't think I appreciated what I had, because it came so naturally. As well as the long jump, I was also good at almost every other event and competed in the multi-events as well, winning my competitions by miles and almost invincible, or so I thought. I broke all the junior records, and at one point held all three English Schools Multi-Event records (the last one was held for 28 years before being broken recently in 2017). Denise Lewis never beat me once when we were juniors.

So you could say I was a lazy athlete. Being an African and coming from a very strict background where both my parents instilled the importance of education first and foremost, I simply thought that athletics was just a temporary plaything and it came second (or even third) to everything else in my life. The order of importance was my Christian life, education, and then athletics. My parents would have freaked out if I came home with anything less than very good grades. Therefore, alongside my athletics career, I studied and got into medical school. They knew nothing about my sporting career until my father got a call one day from his friend to tell him I was competing at the World Championships in Tokyo on television, and was on the news that night. Despite all this, I continued to excel in my career, and I won the European Junior gold medal in 1989 and the silver medal at the Commonwealth Games in Canada in 1994.

After my gold medal win at the European Championships, I was put under immense pressure to try to focus more on my athletics in preparation for the 1992 Olympic Games. One of the hardest things I have ever done was to ask my parents if I could postpone my second year at medical school in order to prepare for the 1992 Barcelona Olympics. My father grudgingly agreed after discussions with the Great Britain team managers and my university, and he also made me promise to spend the year learning other skills, such as shorthand, word processing, and typing. I came 13th in the qualifying rounds at the Olympics, and missed getting into the final by one place, but went on to win the silver medal at the Commonwealth Games.

With all this happening to me at a young age with very little effort, I was on top of the world, and everything seemed fine. However, everything came to a head at the European Junior Championships. I remember vividly that I was entered in both the heptathlon and the long jump. I started with the long jump, which I won by a significant margin, beating the favourite German athlete. This suddenly made me the Golden Girl. I was invited to the press office, the managers were all over me, and the crowd was amazing. The euphoria made me feel loved and important, but how wrong I was. This was going to be my first important lesson about the cruelty of elite sports. The day after winning the long jump, I began the heptathlon. I was on top of the world. No one could stop me. I was winning most of the events, and by the time I came to the final event the next day, I was over 700 points in the lead and almost invincible. The gold medal looked as if it would be mine and I would win double gold. Then along came one of the British team managers just before the last event, which was my worst event, the dreaded 800 m. He gave me some statistics about my closest rival, a German girl who had a personal best in the 800 m that was much better than mine. He told me that if we both ran our personal bests, this girl would win on paper and I would go home with a silver. He got into my psyche and told me I could run much better because I was clearly in shape and doing so well. He then gave me some ridiculous strategy which I innocently tried to follow instead of doing what I normally do. To cut a long story short, it was a disaster. I ended up stepping off the track at the 500 m point because I was so exhausted, I felt that all the other athletes were just pulling away from me, and it was hopeless. I shall never forget the feeling I experienced at that moment. My coach, the British management and coaches, the whole 60,000 odd crowd and other athletes were all shouting at me to get back on the track. I was literally bullied to resume the race, which I did, but I was disqualified anyway for stepping off the track so was awarded no points. Despite that, I still came seventh in the competition, which showed how far ahead I was. Immediately after the race, it was as if I was a different person because neither my coach, nor the management, nor any of the other athletes came to talk to me or console me. Everyone had forgotten that I'd won the gold medal 2 days earlier. Only one coach, Mike, came up to me to console me and said 'Well, you won't do that again, will you! You need to forget about it and put it down to lessons learned and move on'. Although these were words of wisdom, at that time they did not help much. I kept running the race over and over in my head, and I created the image in my mind that I was fat and useless because I just plodded around the track during that 800 m race. That powerful image stayed with me for a long time, and at that point I made up my mind never to do another heptathlon again.

My perception of myself was worsened by various other events that occurred in the following years. This included one day when, while competing in what I believe was the World Cup event, one of the commentators called me a 'stocky' athlete even though I won the event. I took those words to heart, and they compounded the already innate feelings of worthlessness that I had about myself. And so my career continued. Even though I was doing well, I had lost that invincible feeling. I felt judged at every point and I found it difficult to perform easily in front of large crowds. If I did not perform well then, I was a failure, it was not that I was just having a bad day. With hindsight, I would say that I was depressed but I did not know it or understand this. At every point I felt the need to prove myself. I no longer felt the joy I had initially experienced with the sport. I was now just a competitor.

Then one day I met a remarkable person. He was one of the team doctors in one of our international competitions. I think he noticed how I was always putting myself down and speaking negatively about things, and he approached me and asked me why I did this. I tried to give him the 'I am not worthy speech' and he simply laughed at me. This shocked me. I wasn't sure why he was laughing. He told me that I needed to change my mindset about a lot of things and he would be willing to help me do that. He offered me some sports psychology sessions to help me because I was struggling with being around large crowds and people. At this point he had no idea what had happened to me a few years back.

My sessions with Dr Tim were an eye-opener. He had the ability to make me cry at every session, but funnily enough I felt better after each session. The most important thing I learned from him was the phrase 'So What'. First, he made me think about everything I had achieved and was achieving. He said 'so what if people are laughing at you', 'so what if people think you are fat', and 'so what if people think you look ugly'. He told me to remember that it is 'Fat, ugly Yinka that is still beating their butts!'. Then he said that if I really believed I was fat and ugly I should do something about it and stop moaning and feeling sorry for myself. He also told me that the reason why I had not completed that 800 m was not because I was fat, but because I had never trained for it. If I wanted to run a good 800 m then I would need to stop being lazy and train for it. Simple thoughts, but what a revelation! I knew I had to get rid of that European gremlin in my mind so that I could feel good again. The following year I trained for the heptathlon once more, and this time trained for the 800 m. I went to an international competition in Spain, broke the record, and beat everyone with an amazing personal best in the 800 m. I have never done another heptathlon again in my life, but I felt good about having destroyed that particular demon. However, it was not much longer before I gave up the sport because I simply could no longer handle the stress and the public exposure.

Although all of these events happened around 28 years ago, whenever I have to speak about those times I still get very emotional and am affected by that feeling of not being worthy, and of effectively being a 'fake'. I can see now how easy it would have been for anyone else in my position to have become depressed or developed an eating disorder such as bulimia or anorexia. I can also begin to understand how some athletes may end up taking performance-enhancing drugs or undergoing surgery in order to live up to this image that we sometimes have in our heads, and aspire to. I knew a couple of athletes who were caught doping. Those offences came as a shock to me because the athletes looked 'normal' and I could not understand how such nice people could cheat. I also trained with a very lovely German athlete who had previously been on drugs but had never been caught. She explained to me that earlier in her career it was an organizational issue with the German Athletics Federation that if an athlete did not use performance-enhancing drugs, they were not considered to be doing their absolute best. As she grew older, she found herself developing a more mature attitude to this culture that she did not believe in, and was able to distance herself from it. Thus I learned that drug use was clearly evident and rife in the system, and that anyone can be susceptible.

I suppose I never contemplated any of this simply because, as I mentioned earlier, athletics was not at the top of my agenda. Also I think being a Christian helped, and I felt it was morally wrong. Finally, anyone who has ever met my parents would understand that my doing anything illegal or even 'naughty' would probably have signed my death warrant at home, so it was never going to happen. I was a good church-going Christian girl. I didn't smoke, drink alcohol, or fornicate. However, I think that this background also made me very vulnerable and unaware of how unkind and dishonest people can be with their affections. When you are at the top of your game, everyone 'loves' you, but if you make a single mistake or show any kind of human flaw, be prepared for people to show you their true colours.

My son is currently an international athlete and British number one in his event age group, and I was discussing this issue with him. He is very tall and slim but, unlike me, he seems to have put athletics at the top of his agenda in life. He grew up doing sports with me supporting him all the way, in contrast to my parents' attitude. He lives and breathes athletics. As a parent, I would prefer his studies to come first, but I would like to think that I have always allowed all my children to follow their passions. I know that my son takes his protein shakes and potions, but he has told me that as an elite athlete he knows that it is his responsibility to check that none of the ingredients in the shakes include banned substances. I asked him why he drinks these shakes and if he would ever be tempted to take banned substances to enhance his performance, or if he has ever been offered such things, and his response surprised me. Although he said it jokingly, his words were clear: 'Mum, if I got caught with anything you would kill me'. I laughed, but that statement did not make me as happy as his next words. He went on to tell me that although athletics was very important to him, he did not think the risk of taking illegal substances was worth it. He said it was like robbing a bank. All robbers perform a heist with the initial certainty that they will never be caught, but when they are caught they must then suffer the judicial consequences. It is exactly the same with illegal substances. Either you get caught by the sporting body, or your health will eventually suffer the consequences. That for me was one of the most mature things I have ever heard him say. He also went on to explain that he took the protein shakes and other concoctions in order to meet the nutritional requirements of his training more quickly. This makes absolute sense, and is consistent with the behaviours of so many millennium children who need everything done at the speed of light. No one writes letters anymore – everything is done by email. They want to communicate faster, they want instant fast food, they want love at the click of a mouse button or via Tinder or some app, without having to wait for it. So here, instead of having 10 eggs in a blender in the morning, my son can get the same protein by adding one teaspoonful of powder to his protein shake.

To conclude, I would say that it is important for clinicians to understand the physical, psychological, and environmental factors relating to individuals when considering the links between exercise, self-image, and clinical conditions, especially psychological and mental health conditions. Factors that need to be considered include the level at which the person practises the sport or exercise, the reasons why they do so or the enjoyment they derive from that exercise or sport, the importance of the sport on the agenda of their life, the personal support they receive, and finally what I believe is most important of all, their personality and how they respond to challenges. For someone like me, because I naturally tend to have low self-esteem and a poor opinion of myself and my abilities, I constantly need people like Dr Tim to remind me that I am worthy, to prevent me from living a depressive life of self-condemnation. This has continued through my life, and you will notice that I have a lot of qualifications because I still feel the need to prove my worth, while suffering from something called 'imposter syndrome'. My son, on the other hand, is very clear about his abilities and about the fact that he deserves to be where he is, in the top ranks. He will not be influenced by others or have his sense of worth measured by other people's opinions or the number of letters after his name. Some may call this arrogance, but I would like to think that it is because he has grown up as a confident young man who knows that he is loved and will not be judged on account of his choices.

In view of my life and the challenges I have faced, over the years I have decided to dedicate my time to developing and motivating others. I am in the process of writing my first book, which I hope will inspire others to love themselves and remember that they have worth even when others fail to appreciate them. If that is my only lasting legacy, all the pain and trauma will have been worthwhile, as they can help others who may be in similar situations.

Index